Praise

The Complete M

COLIN CAMPBELL

Denny Waxman offers an informed account of the macrobiotic dietary lifestyle that has been pivotal to a new way of thinking about diet and health during the past half century. This is the "go-to" book for this way of eating.

—T. Colin Campbell, Ph.D.
Jacob Gould Schurman Professor Emeritus
of Nutritional Biochemistry
Cornell University

NEAL BARNARD

To a physician, macrobiotics is impressive. I have seen many patients who faced daunting medical problems for which mainstream approaches were simply ineffective, and who used basic macrobiotic principles to regain their health and vitality. This book is your key to understanding these principles and putting them to work. Denny Waxman is a leader in the world of macrobiotics and, in this simple guide, he shares his wisdom and practical tips with you. You will love the foods that will become part of your life, and you will love how you feel. In short order, this book will change your life.

—Neal D. Barnard, M.D.
President, Physicians Committee for Responsible Medicine

CRAIG BORTEN

Denny has been changing the world of conventional thinking regarding health for the past 40 years and has had the courage to stand tall against the powerful forces of industry and government . . . my kind of character!

—Craig Borten
Academy Award Nominee, Best Original Screenplay,
Dallas Buyers Club

STEWART RAFFILL

Our bodies are amazing machines that require an intricate balance for good health. Denny Waxman has deciphered this amazing riddle and knows how to bring us back to homeostasis through a combination of ancient and modern dietary applications. He is a gifted healer and I have had the pleasure of seeing him transform and heal many people—including myself.

—Stewart Raffill
Hollywood writer/director

STACEY CANTOR-ADKINS

Denny Waxman has synthesized the essence of macrobiotics in 7 steps that are easy to remember and put into practice. Many of the recommendations that come from time-tested traditional wisdom are now being confirmed by evidence-based medicine, such as the use of probiotic-rich, naturally-fermented foods, chewing food well to begin digestion, sitting to eat in a low-stress environment, and consuming a mainly plant-based, whole foods diet. The steps that Denny elucidates will become like a mantra to those who follow them, such as sit down to eat without doing other things, and have a grain and vegetable dish with each meal. Macrobiotics, as instructed by Denny Waxman, helped me to recover my health, and it will help you also, to live the "big life."

—Stacey Cantor-Adkins, M.D.
Functional Medicine and Nutrition

MARTHA CLAYTON COTTRELL

This book is a treasure! It is a great handbook, packed with information and instructions, if followed, will result in the enhancement of one's Health of Mind, Body and Spirit.

—Martha Clayton Cottrell, M.D.

ANH-HUONG NGUYEN

Denny Waxman's practice and teaching on macrobiotics carry in them the essence of Buddhist teachings on interbeing, happiness, and compassion.

Through his message and conviction that personal health is the basis for planetary health, I see in him a truly engaged Buddhist.

—Anh-Huong Nguyen
Meditation Teacher
Author of "Walking Meditation"

JEFFREY DUBB, M.D.

After graduating from the University of Chicago Medical School, I worked as a research physician for a large multinational pharmaceutical company. I was steeped in the scientific method and the value of clinical trials. I thought that for every disease, there must be a medication that could help the condition.

However, after having the good fortune of marrying a woman who was macrobiotic and had studied with Denny Waxman for many years, I have come to appreciate the power that lifestyle and food have over one's health. I now realize that a macrobiotic diet offers the possibility for a deeper level of health than is available with the dietary recommendations of conventional medicine.

I am grateful to Denny for his depth of knowledge and his great experience in applying macrobiotic principles to human health. His teachings have allowed me to enjoy a happier and more vigorous life.

—Jeffrey Dubb, M.D.
Philadelphia

TOM MONTE

Anyone who reads this book and follows Denny Waxman's advice will experience better health, greater happiness, and deeper insight into the meaning of life.

—Tom Monte, author of
The Complete Guide to Natural Healing

JESSICA PORTER

Denny Waxman's system of teaching is flexible, unique, and refreshing. *The Complete Macrobiotic Diet* is a really cool book.

—Jessica Porter, author of
The Hip Chicks Guide to Macrobiotics:
A Philosophy for Achieving a Radiant Mind
and a Fabulous Body

THE
Complete
Macrobiotic
DIET

7 STEPS
TO FEEL FABULOUS, LOOK VIBRANT, AND THINK CLEARLY

DENNY WAXMAN WITH **SUSAN WAXMAN**

PREFACE BY MICHIO KUSHI

PEGASUS BOOKS
NEW YORK LONDON

THE COMPLETE MACROBIOTIC DIET

Pegasus Books LLC
80 Broad Street, 5th Floor
New York, NY 10004

Interior design by Maria Fernandez

ISBN: 978-1-60598-666-1

10 9 8 7 6 5 4 3 2 1

Printed in the United States of America
Distributed by W. W. Norton & Company, Inc.

In memory of our friend

Mona Schwartz,

whose encouragement and spirit have guided this book.

DISCLAIMER

The information contained in this book is intended solely to provide guidance and to increase the reader's awareness about the dietary and lifestyle practices that can create lasting health.

If you suspect that you have a medical problem, we urge you to seek competent medical help and be aware that a second medical opinion is often the best course to achieve the best outcome for any particular condition.

CONTENTS

PREFACE
BY MICHIO KUSHI

Humanity faces unparalleled opportunities and challenges as the new century unfolds. The world is unified more than ever through the Internet, cell phones, and other new technologies. At the same time, the threat of terrorism and nuclear blackmail, the outbreak of new viral diseases and epidemics, and the spread of cancer, heart disease, and other chronic ills are at an all-time high. If we don't destroy ourselves through war and sickness, our children and grandchildren may inherit a globally warmed planet that is too extreme to inhabit.

For the last half-century, macrobiotics has been in the forefront of the movement to promote personal and planetary health and peace. Derived from the traditional Greek words for "great life," macrobiotics encourages people to take responsibility for their own health and happiness by harmonizing with Nature and the cosmos. The most effective way to do this is to eat a balanced natural-foods diet, centered on whole grains and vegetables, in harmony with the seasons, the climate, and other environmental factors.

The value of this approach is now almost universally accepted. In its food guidelines for the American people, the U.S. government officially promotes whole grains as the foundation of a healthy diet. The newest version of the Food Guide Pyramid, released in 2005, calls for brown rice, millet, whole wheat, and other grains to be the center of every meal.

The benefits of a macrobiotic diet are becoming increasingly recognized. At Harvard Medical School, cardiovascular researchers report that people eating a macrobiotic diet for an average of two years have virtually no risk of coronary heart disease, the major cause of death in modern society. Scientists at Tulane University in New Orleans, Louisiana and the National Tumor Institute in Milan, Italy report that a macrobiotic diet may help prevent or control cancer. Researchers at the New England Medical Center in Boston report that macrobiotic women process estrogen better than others and this may explain their low incidence of breast cancer. The National Cancer Institute has approved the start of clinical trials on the macrobiotic approach to cancer after reviewing several of 76 medically documented recoveries compiled by researchers for the National Institutes of Health.

Other medical studies have shown that a macrobiotic way of eating is beneficial for improving childhood nutrition, reducing violent and aggressive behavior among young juvenile offenders, controlling T-cells in young adults with AIDS, improving geriatric and psychiatric health, and reducing multiple chemical sensitivities.

According to environmentalists, a macrobiotic-oriented diet will benefit the earth as well as the people it sustains.

Growing grains and vegetables as our staple crops instead of animal foods reduces our dependence on fossil fuels, chemicals, and other toxins, enriches the fertility of the soil, and results in cleaner air and water.

Over the years, Denny Waxman has been one of my closest students and associates and has served in the forefront of this health revolution. He founded Essene, the pioneer natural-foods store in Philadelphia, in the late 1960s and organized seminars on diet and health in the 1970s. In the early 1980s, he helped Anthony J. Satillaro, M.D., the president of Methodist Hospital in Philadelphia, recover from terminal cancer. The story was featured in the *Saturday Evening Post, Life* Magazine, and later in a best-selling book *Recalled by Life* and has helped to popularize macrobiotics around the world. At the Strengthening Health Institute that he founded in the 1990s, Denny has developed a simple, practical approach to macrobiotic education that focuses on seven steps to better health.

In *The Complete Macrobiotic Diet*, Denny distills the essence of macrobiotic principles and teachings. He presents his seven steps in a clear, concise way that can be readily understood and practiced. Seasoned with insights and humor from his personal experience, counseling practice, and global travels, the book offers a compass to maintaining health, happiness, and freedom. A wealth of practical information, including lists of recommended foods, basic recipes, and meal suggestions, helps the reader get started.

Thanks to Denny and a remarkable generation of macrobiotic teachers, counselors, and natural-food cooks, the seeds of a healthy, peaceful world community have been planted.

The Complete Macrobiotic Diet is a passport to a healthier, more harmonious life.

Michio Kushi
Brookline, Massachusetts
February 4, 2006

Michio Kushi is the leader of the international macrobiotic community. The Smithsonian Institution recognized his pioneering contribution to the modern organic natural-foods movement; complementary and alternative medicine; and peace education by establishing a permanent Kushi Family Collection on Macrobiotics at the National Museum of American History in Washington, D.C.

TESTIMONIALS

"No disease that can be treated by diet should be treated with any other means."

—Maimonides

"He who has health has hope, and he who has hope has everything."

—Arabic Proverb

Facts and lessons learned from guiding Dr. Anthony Sattilaro to health from terminal prostate cancer.

Dr. Anthony Sattilaro was the president of Methodist Hospital in Philadelphia. In May 1978, he was diagnosed with terminal prostate cancer that had spread to his whole body. In August 1979, the cancer was gone. After further medical tests in 1981, his doctors declared him to be in complete remission.

My first client, Mona Schwartz, was at my house when Dr. Sattilaro came for a consultation with me. He had found out about me by accident after picking up some hitchhikers who were cooks at my summer camp. When he left, Mona asked me to look after him the same way that I had done with her. My impetus to look after him personally the best way that I could was at her urging. I invited Dr. Sattilaro to eat at my house every day and guided him with food recommendations: more of this, less of that, focus here, etc. I helped him to develop the skill to make decisions that support health.

He attended lectures and seminars about macrobiotic eating and never missed a cooking class. The macrobiotic community in Philadelphia at the time also fully supported and encouraged him throughout the recovery process. I introduced him to Michio Kushi, who also became a part of his recovery.

Dr. Sattilaro documented his recovery at every step. His story was published first by the Saturday Evening Post and *Life* magazine and later in his book *Recalled by Life*, which became an international best seller. The articles are available to read on my website.

I learned many lessons about what it meant to me to be a counselor through guiding Dr. Sattilaro. I gained a deep confidence in my own ability to help people create lasting health, especially when I had the ability to guide them closely. Terminal illness means modern medicine does not have the understanding or the technology to help or reverse it. I have personally observed hundreds of people reverse terminal illness. My life's work has evolved into doing what medicine can't. Hippocrates, the father of western medicine, recommended diet and lifestyle practices as the best medicine.

Macrobiotics is about the cultivation of spiritual, mental, and physical health. Even in sickness, the emphasis is still on the cultivation of health. As we increase health, sickness naturally diminishes in our life. "Recovery" in macrobiotics is a spiritual revolution where we learn how to guide and create our own health and life.

Active participants in their own recovery always do better. They take the time to find out what to do and get involved with creating their own health. The journey toward health is an energizing adventure, and education is a very important part of the process.

Proper support is vital for any recovery; support is more than approval, it is a collaboration. Real support means "let's do this together" and moves us toward our goal of health.

In my experience, there are three common points that lead to recovery. The first is finding good guidance. The second is education through books and seminars. The third is putting together a good support team. People who make recovery their number one priority are the ones who recover.

The following testimonials are from some of my clients. People accomplished seemingly miraculous transformations after accurately and vigorously applying the principles in this book. Some people have chosen to combine these principles with traditional medical treatments while others have used them alone. In either case, please consult with your medical professional before making these dietary and lifestyle modifications. It is also important to find a medical professional who will support you in your healing journey. I am sure you will be inspired from these experiences. Our bodies have amazing healing abilities when we treat them with love, care, and respect.

THE STORY OF STACEY L. CANTOR-ADKINS, *M.D.*

Macrobiotics saved my life. Eighteen years ago, I was incapacitated with Chronic Fatigue Syndrome, from which I had been suffering for fourteen years. Then I discovered macrobiotics and Denny Waxman, and my fortunes began to change. He showed me that my diet and lifestyle contributed to my illness and how, by reversing these factors, I could heal myself. With a lot of hard work, I was able to reclaim my health and my life.

Three years later, Denny then guided me through a natural and healthy pregnancy and childbirth. Afterwards, he counseled me in raising my child according to the macrobiotic lifestyle.

I began to study with Denny Waxman as soon as I began counseling with him. I completed the two-year Macrobiotic Counselor Training Program at the Strengthening Health Institute and continued with the Graduate Studies Program. I can say from my vast experience that Denny is an educator, counselor, and motivator par excellence. With his keen intuition and his mastery of macrobiotic theory, he offers amazingly effective solutions and recommendations. He clearly explains how macrobiotics is a way of understanding the universal laws of Nature, so we can make better choices about how to direct our lives. His teachings extend far beyond individual self-healing, however. He teaches how this universal macrobiotic understanding can also be used to create practical approaches to healing environmental, societal, and global ills.

Denny Waxman is a serious thinker and true visionary with a large world view, working to promote personal and planetary health. He is the kind of inspirational leader of which the world is in short supply. He is uniquely poised to lead us through these troubled times, by showing us how we can rediscover our common sense and intuition to live to our full potential and create a more peaceful and joyous world.

THE STORY OF NOELLE ARTHERHOLT, *FUND ACCOUNTANT AND MOM*

It has been three years since my diagnosis with a Cavernous Sinus Meningioma, basically a benign brain tumor in a not so good location. I was 33 and had 10 weeks left in my 2nd pregnancy. I went for several opinions on how best to address my situation and was given opinions ranging from surgery to radiation. The consistency in the opinions regarded the permanency of symptoms of double vision and numbness of my tongue and the right side of my face if I did not go for treatment. I truly felt in my heart that I could heal myself and thus began my journey to find an advocate.

From the moment I met Denny, I felt comfortable and confident in his knowledge and advice on what I should adapt in my life. By furthermore attending the Strengthening Health Institute, I learned the skills I needed, from the fundamentals of macrobiotics, to food preparation and menu planning.

All my symptoms have since disappeared and although doctors advised me not to have any more children on chance of my tumor being hormone related, I did have a third child. It was a beautiful pregnancy with no complications or symptoms. I am grateful for all that you continue to teach me as I evolve on my macrobiotic journey amidst the wonderful chaos of my house with three healthy young children.

"Each patient carries his own doctor inside him."
—Norman Cousins

THE STORY OF JOHN AND TOINI WILLIAMS, *SENIOR MAINTENANCE REPAIR*

Four days after our wedding, I was diagnosed with testicular cancer. In support of my desire to try a natural healing approach, my wife Toini got some books on macrobiotics. We discovered Denny Waxman through *Recalled By Life* by Dr. Anthony Sattilaro. We went to see Denny and began a journey that transformed our lives and how we view health.

I strictly followed Denny's dietary recommendations for two years. The tumor shrank, and the pain went away. I felt so good, I went off the diet and the cancer spread fast and suddenly. Cat scans and other tests revealed that I had stage 3 testicular seminoma. To my great fortune, two doctors on staff at Methodist Hospital in Philadelphia (where Dr. Sattilaro worked) were macrobiotic themselves and were a great encouragement to me as I underwent the chemo and radiation that was to follow. Once the chemo and radiation halted the cancer, I was told that any more chemo would kill me. After surgery, I decided to seriously return to the diet to heal. One huge side effect of all the treatment was that I would not be able to father children.

When we told Denny about it, he assured us that within two years of following his dietary and lifestyle recommendations, I could eliminate all the toxins and reverse the effect of the chemo and radiation. In just a little over two years time, our first son was born on Christmas morning. Another son and two daughters were to follow, our youngest born to us when we were forty-four years old.

At a newborn-baby checkup with our third child, the doctor asked about my medical history. When I told him about my bout with stage 3 testicular cancer and the treatments, he looked confused. He though I had undergone treatment AFTER my wife was pregnant and when he found out, he was amazed. He stated that men who go through the treatments for this cancer cannot father children.

Although healing from cancer and fathering children when I was told I wouldn't be able to are dramatic aspects to this story, the everyday benefits are what make up a life of transformation. Denny's intuition and recommendations, even over the phone, are invaluable for health crises. It is uncanny how he can recommend a drink or dish that will eliminate physical problems. Our seventeen-year-old daughter recently said she feels confident she can deal with most everyday illness herself using her knowledge of the diet. I feel truly blessed to know Denny Waxman, and grateful that he dedicated his life to the study of macrobiotics and strengthening health.

THE STORY OF NANCY WOLFSON-MOCHE, *NOURISHMENT EDUCATOR, COUNSELOR, AND BLOGGER*

Prior to getting married, I sought help from Denny for a few different conditions that were completely resolved after following his recommendations. When I got married at forty-two, I began trying to conceive. After several months, and after learning I was not eligible for any hi-tech fertility treatments due to my elevated FSH level, I went to see Denny. I worked closely with him and over the course of a year my FSH dropped by 25 points. Soon after that, I became pregnant at age forty-four. Denny guided me through a healthy pregnancy and I worked closely with him during the first few years of my daughter's life. He was always responsive, open, and highly professional. Over the following five years we worked closely to tweak and fine-tune my diet and lifestyle. With Denny's guidance and support, I was able to have a second baby at the age of fifty-one.

Denny is a brilliant, generous, patient, and wise counselor, teacher, and thinker.

"The doctor of the future will no longer treat the human frame with drugs, but rather will cure and prevent disease with nutrition."

—Thomas Edison

THE STORY OF SIGRID GEERLINGS, *SENIOR ASSOCIATE FOR NEW THEME INC.*

I think I might be the medical version of an X-file, which rather thrills me. I'm referring of course to the TV show about FBI cases concerning unexplained phenomena, filed away and forgotten. Similarly, my carcinoma's disappearance thanks to macrobiotics will not be included in any medical statistics or even written up in my personal medical file as such; it was deemed unexplainable by my surgeon. Yet the truth about the way the body can heal itself is out there.

About two years ago, I had really bad migraines. My husband had been macrobiotic twenty years earlier and told me to call Denny Waxman. When I called Denny to make an appointment I mentioned that my son, who was four at the time, had speech delay and a number of other vague global delay symptoms that were deemed either extremely serious or totally transient, depending on which professional gave what opinion. My son and I both went to see Denny, and in both our cases we were helped enormously by making just the basic changes. My son improved overnight!

Shortly after that, a mammogram and a needle biopsy showed that I had DCIS, or Ductal Carcinoma In Situ, which is a stage 0 cancer, with III grade cell necrosis. My medical treatment options ranged from a full mastectomy of both breasts, and medication for life since I was "lucky" enough to have the right kind of cancer, to a lumpectomy with radiation. When I told one of my doctors that I wanted to try macrobiotics for 6 months, he allowed that for that period of time, my condition probably wouldn't become life-threatening, so I felt quite safe to delay and hopefully avoid medical intervention. The very next day, I received a call that they had looked at the biopsy slides again and found a suspicious-looking spot that might be interpreted as an inflammatory cancer. They urged me to at least get a lumpectomy right away. I thought they tried to scare me into going the medical route. At my most cynical, I thought they wanted me on board because I would make a pretty good candidate for their HER2 clinical study, being fairly young and healthy. Instead, I went back to Denny.

I took the Strengthening Health Intensive, which changed my whole being. From that weekend on, I cooked gorgeous and delicious food, took walks, rubbed my skin, tried to meditate, and received amazing Shiatsu massages. I discharged.

About 4 months after I took the Strengthening Health Intensive, my breast started to hurt. Denny and I suspected that the metal marker left at the site of the biopsy was causing the pain. I needed surgery to have it removed. The tissue my surgeon took out was completely clear of DCIS.

Before the surgery, my surgeon said: Hey, if it's gone, we'll say macrobiotics cured it. After the results came back, she said: I can't say macrobiotics cured it. Maybe the needle biopsy removed it all, maybe it went away by itself. She Scullied me and I'm sure the word "macrobiotics" never made it into my medical file; it's an unexplained disappearance of cancer.

I believe . . .

THE STORY OF STEVE GITTELMAN, *WOODWORKER* AND SUSAN HEINEMAN, *FINANCIAL EDUCATION & T'AI CHI INSTRUCTOR*

My partner Steve was diagnosed with Alzheimer's at age fifty-seven. After the diagnosis, he agreed to change his diet. We decided to explore the macrobiotic path and began counseling with Denny Waxman. Steve followed the recommendations and hoped the food would help him.

Denny Waxman's counseling during those years was crucial for both Steve and me. I credit Denny's guidance and the diet for bringing stability and a sense of confidence and well-being into Steve's life. Denny gave us purpose, direction, clarity, and hope.

As a result of working with Denny Waxman, the following changes took place for Steve:

- Chronic dandruff gone
- Lowered and normalized cholesterol
- Gradual, effortless 50-pound weight loss, balancing to his ideal 160
- Stabilized blood sugar levels
- Improvement in mood, attitude, clarity of thinking, freedom of movement, overall well-being

THE STORY OF JACK SCHULTZ, *CEO/PRESIDENT JERSEY SHORE STEEL: GREEN STEEL MANUFACTURER*

Five years ago, I underwent a total knee replacement. My wife, Carole, is very careful concerning her diet and she suggested that I exercise the same discipline concerning my diet as well. Under the direction of Denny Waxman, and with the help of his wife, Susan, and Carole, a healing diet was recommended.

I remained in Philadelphia for six weeks, doing my exercises and watching my diet. After the initial six weeks, my surgeon and his staff were so pleased with my progress that they felt it was unnecessary for me to return to Philadelphia for the normal twelve-week post-op checkup. When I returned to Williamsport to continue my therapy, the therapist inquired where I had the operation since she had never seen anyone recover as quickly as I had. I attribute my quick recovery, my loss of forty pounds, and the fact that I was able to get off the pain medication so quickly, to the discipline I followed concerning my diet.

ACKNOWLEDGMENTS

This book represents a major portion of my life, and these acknowledgments are for all of the people who have helped me and are therefore a part of it.

Without my parents, Anna and Herman Waxman, I would not be able to offer this book. I acknowledge them with deepest respect and appreciation.

To Michio and Aveline Kushi, my spiritual parents, who have spent their lives teaching macrobiotics and spreading it throughout the world. They have given me endless inspiration, encouragement, and personal guidance.

To my teachers, George and Lima Ohsawa, Herman and Cornelia Aihara, Shizuko Yamamoto, and William Dufty, who have dedicated their lives to macrobiotics and gave us this powerful legacy.

To my brother, Howard, who shared the dream of macrobiotics and Essene with me.

To my children: Nathan, Joe, Naomi, Alisa, Madeline, Amy, Zoe, Andrew, Natasha, and Sam, their significant others, and my grandchildren Isiah, Sienna, and Thomas, who brighten my life.

To Jared, Barbara, Julie, and Lauren, who have become an important part of my life.

To Mona Schwartz, my friend and mentor, who encouraged me to develop macrobiotics in a more broad and spiritual direction.

To Ellen Brodkey, my close and endearing friend, who has worked long and hard to make this book possible.

To Stephanie Bartusis, whose persistence, insight, and bright enthusiasm helped bring this new addition to life.

To my wife, Susan, who shares this book, my life, and my dreams. Susan cooks like an angel and her caring, loving nature comes through in every dish she makes. I hope you experience it through her recipes.

To Takashi Yoshikawa, who has guided us and helped us greatly to broaden and deepen our understanding of *ki*, which we have used to strengthen the health and lives of all of those we have been privileged to help.

To our publisher, Claiborne Hancock, for believing in us and making this book possible. To Jamie Armfield for introducing us to Claiborne.

To our dear friends Doug FitzSimons, Don and Mary Marti, and Helen Stevenson, who have played a significant role in our lives.

To our friends and associates: Bill Tara, Murray Snyder, Bill Spear, Judith Flohr, Melanie Waxman, Chico and Geninha Varatojo, Rik Vermuyten, Michel Matsuda, Patrick Riley, Michel Abehsera, Michael Kessler, Simon Brown, Norio, Larry and Phiya Kushi, Gary Flaxenburg, Rod and Peggy House, and Gabor Szalontay, with whom we have shared many macrobiotic adventures.

There are so many friends who have become part of our lives through SHI. All have been parts of our efforts to create a more healthy, peaceful world in different ways. To name just a few: Warren Kramer, Michelle Nemer, Tom Spring, Robert and Kathryn Burdick, Russ and Nancy Merrick, Phil and Susan Harris, Carole and Jack Schultz, Stewart Raffill and Diane Kirman, Ruth Ann and Jeffrey Dubb, Richard Epstein and Luanne Thomas, Carol Tamburino, Bill Bergman, Lori Eckstein, Deborah Albanese, Ralph Jenkins, Carlotta Lala, Natasha Novoselova, Jeff Silberman and Sigrid Geerlings, Mary McCabe, Loretta Lombardi, Kirin McElwain, Traci Opdahl, Peggy Pastore, Georgene Pijut, Theresa Schultz, Kathy Duggan, Gina Compello, Stephen Prudente, and all of our friends at Essene, without whom our dream of building a school could not have been realized.

To our many other friends, too numerous to name, but you know who you are and I thank you.

—Denny Waxman

In addition to all of the people listed previously, I would like to share my personal acknowledgments.

A very special thank you to my parents, Barbara and Jared Schwalm, for their love, nurturance, and wisdom, which has given me the foundation to help become the person I am today.

To all of my family, especially my sister and brother-in-law, Julie and Loren Wolgemuth, Howard Waxman and Janet Jaffe, my children, grandchildren, and Ichi. I love you all!

A special thank you to my dear friend Ralph Jenkins, who is always there for me, introduced me to macrobiotics, and got me started on this journey.

To my dear friends, Mona Schwartz and Ellen Brodkey, who have encouraged, mentored, and helped me to develop as a teacher and as a woman.

A huge thank you to Kirin McElwain for all of her hard work, dedication, inspiration, love, and most of all friendship. To Stephanie Bartusis for her patience, hard work, inspiration and organizing us, which is not an easy task! Thank you both for helping us to bring our voice to paper.

Thank you to all of my friends, who know who they are, and more importantly I know who they are. Thank you for putting up with me, waiting for me to get ready, for loving and supporting me, and sharing good times.

Finally I would like to thank my husband, Denny Waxman, whose insight into philosophy, health, diet, and lifestyle is brilliant. Thank you for loving, teaching, and encouraging me. Thank you for the opportunity to be a part of this book and finally express my work and knowledge on a much broader level. My hope is that many people read and become inspired with this book and our work.

—Susan Waxman

FOREWORD

"Take care of your body with steadfast fidelity. The
soul must see things through these eyes alone, and
if they are dim, the whole world is clouded."
                                    —Johann Wolfgang von Goethe

This book represents more than four decades of my life. Since
I first tasted brown rice in 1967, I have been committed to
understanding the principles of macrobiotics through study,
practice, counseling, and teaching. I have used the profound
wisdom contained in these principles to transform my own
life, to help raise healthy children, to guide thousands of clients back to health, and to improve the health of countless
others who have attended my seminars over the years. My goal
has been, and continues to be, to find new ways to simplify
and clarify these fundamental principles so they can be understood easily and practiced accurately by anyone interested in
this way of life. Good health is our birthright and our heritage
and ought to be available to everyone.

People want better health, but they don't know how to
achieve it. There is simply too much information available,

and it changes at too rapid a pace to be reliable. What's worse, this information, on which many people base their health practices, often turns out to be conflicting. My first book, *Ten Steps to Strengthening Health*, published in 1997, was written with the intention of cutting through all the confusion. However, the world has changed rapidly and profoundly since then and, while the principles of macrobiotics are bedrock and don't change, the ways in which we put these principles into practice must. If we fail to adapt to the ever-changing conditions around us, through ignorance or neglect, our health will suffer. *Seven Steps to Strengthening Health* was conceived as a guide to the changed world in which we find ourselves. Please don't be misled by it being called the "Seven Steps." Logic might tell you that there are three fewer steps, but actually there are two additional ones. The ten steps were preserved but restructured into five steps and then two new steps were added.

We can all make better choices every day, under any circumstances, if we understand what constitutes a good choice. The Strengthening Health Approach to Macrobiotics, which stresses an orderly approach to eating and living, is based on creating good eating habits, healthful food choices, and a way of life that nourishes the spirit. Both books came into existence because of the frustration I felt at seeing people make often-heroic efforts to improve their health, yet not achieve the hoped-for results. I have tested and observed the value of the Strengthening Health principles over many years, and I am no longer amazed when I see a person change dramatically after just two or three weeks of following these principles.

"Tradition is a guide and not a jailer."

—W. Somerset Maugham

Macrobiotic practice developed from the common understanding and experience of the world's long-standing civilizations. We have inherited a great wealth from these civilizations. History is our guidebook. Science now continues to validate history. The personal, social, and environmental benefits of a healthful diet and lifestyle have already been scientifically proven. It will not be long before science confirms the value of a life lived in the spirit of gratitude and appreciation. The way to a healthy future for all is to combine history and science.

The Complete Macrobiotic Diet uses the word "diet" in its original meaning as a way of life. This book provides the tools, practical applications, and understanding to live a healthy, and enjoyable, plant-based a way of life.

INTRODUCTION

"The first wealth is health."
—Ralph Waldo Emerson

February 10, 1969 was the turning point of my life. It was the first day of my macrobiotic practice. A lot has happened since that day; a lot had happened before that day. I'd like to tell you about some of it.

I didn't embark on this way of life because of illness or because I saw it as a way of increasing my energy, but because I was dissatisfied with my life. I had always had more than enough energy, perhaps too much, and my head was filled with ideas. My problem was figuring out what to do with all that vitality and all those ideas—in other words, what to do with my life.

I was graduated from high school in 1967, at the age of seventeen. Rather than work at a job I knew I wouldn't enjoy, I decided to try college. Six months into the first semester, I found my classes so boring and so meaningless that I dropped out to study on my own. That plan didn't work out either. The books I read depressed me even more. Many of them spoke of the glorious life and greatly enhanced abilities you could achieve through the development of your consciousness. Though their approaches differed, on one point the authors were all in agreement. In order to move in this direction, a teacher was required. But none of these books told me where to find one.

It was during this somewhat dark and restless period of my life that I first heard the word "macrobiotics." A friend's older brother used it in the process of describing a way of getting high by eating just brown rice. Of course, that is hardly what macrobiotics is all about, but it caught my attention because of my own disastrous diet. I was a junk-food addict. I ate meat only if it was between two slices of bread and I hated vegetables. I lived on sandwiches, pizza, cookies, candy, cake, and soft drinks. Breakfast was my most substantial meal of the day, and it consisted of a toasted bagel with butter and a coke. I will say, in my defense, that around this time I did notice that I was eating more and more junk food and feeling less and less satisfied—so the thought of eating brown rice and feeling better was quite appealing. Eager as I was to learn more about macrobiotics, no one I asked could tell me anything. My own stubbornness made me persist in the search and, eventually, a book appeared that would change my life.

THE UNIFYING PRINCIPLE

I came home one day to a house I shared with a group of friends in Philadelphia, to find a copy of *You Are All San-puku* by George Ohsawa, the "father" of macrobiotics, on my bed. To this day, I have no idea how it got there. The book, which has an extensive introduction by William Dufty, one of

Ohsawa's star students, transported me. It was the first book I'd ever read from beginning to end in one sitting and everything I had been searching for was in it. Ohsawa believed that we have the capacity to change our lives—that it is out of our daily diet and lifestyle, things over which we have some measure of control, that we create our lives, for better or worse.

Ohsawa's book introduced me to the ancient eastern concept of Yin Yang, the principle of balance, harmony, and change. He called it the "unique" or "unifying principle" because it explained both the unity and diversity of all things. In the Eastern way of thinking, all of life has this dual nature.

I was more than ready to try something new. I went out the next day and bought brown rice, sea salt, and mu tea (a kind of Eastern herbal drink), and rushed home to cook my first meal. The taste was interesting—not good, not bad—but I felt wonderful and inspired. And so it was that I began my first 10-day rice fast as described by Ohsawa in his book. I didn't know it at the time, but this was also the beginning of a new and wonderful life. Nor did I know I was having my first lesson in the unifying principle. And I most certainly didn't know that trouble was on the way.

The third day of my new regimen found me in the supermarket, buying a half-gallon of ice cream, a box of graham crackers, and a quart of orange juice. By the time I reached the checkout counter, I'd eaten most everything in the cart. To say that I was disappointed and confused is to understate the case. I knew in my heart that this philosophy and way of life were what I had been looking for—but, obviously, the diet was impossible. I had to find someone who knew more about macrobiotics.

As luck would have it, one day while I was having lunch in a health-food store, a guy with a very intense look about him walked in. For some reason, I thought he might be macrobiotic and I was right. He told me he had come to Philadelphia to change the consciousness level of the city by opening a macrobiotic restaurant and that, yes, he was open to having a partner. A few days later, Stanley and I leased space in an underground mall called Sansom Village. That was on February 10, 1969.

Shortly afterwards, Stanley introduced me to Rod and Peggy House, two of Philadelphia's early macrobiotic friends, who gave me some invaluable dietary advice. The first thing they did was to suggest that I eat vegetables along with my brown rice, a change that made all the difference. That night, I ate my last steak sandwich and made my personal vow to practice the macrobiotic way of life. With the help and guidance of Rod and Peggy, I found the diet easy to follow and the food delicious and satisfying. What I learned from my earlier, unsuccessful attempt to change my diet became the central point of what I would teach others—the importance of flexibility and common sense coupled with the understanding that change can happen gradually or it can happen in a flash.

A few days after we signed the lease, Stanley and I learned that the space wasn't zoned for a restaurant, which forced us to change our plans. We decided instead to open a food market with a lunch counter. We called it Essene Macrobiotic Supply. Shortly before the store opened, Michio Kushi, a world-renowned authority on macrobiotics and a former student of George Ohsawa's, came to Philadelphia to give a two-day seminar. I was one of the two hundred and seventy-five people who had gathered to greet him, and when I asked if he had any advice for our store he said, "Keep it clean. If it's not clean, it's not macrobiotic. I have seen many stores and restaurants that are not macrobiotic although they claim to be."

I couldn't believe that these were his words of wisdom. Keep it clean? Once again, I didn't understand the importance of what I was hearing. But I kept the store clean; and over the years, when people would comment on its cleanliness and tell me how wonderful it was to shop in such a place, I would thank them and think of Michio with gratitude.

We opened to the public on March 21, 1969 with six different products on the shelves, all of them in brown paper bags. People thought we were selling dog food. We weren't disheartened. We continued to sell packaged grains from the shelves, adding some prepared food at the counter—cooked brown rice, miso soup, sautéed vegetables, raw salad, home-baked bread with apple or peanut butter, organic apple juice, fresh carrot juice, and bancha tea.

Apparently, customers liked what we had to offer. They returned, bringing friends. Business grew, and we were able to fill the shelves with a variety of products. Our customers were curious. They wanted to know more about this mysterious food and the philosophy behind it. I told them about the wonders of eating grains and vegetables and about the harm that animal food, dairy, sugar, and refined foods were inflicting on their bodies and minds. Some were interested; others were not and left. I decided to stop talking before we lost them all! Something good came out of this, however. I noticed that our regular customers began to change. They looked different—fresher, younger, more attractive. And these changes happened in a very short time.

PERSONAL CHANGES AND STUDIES

I was changing too. I had even more energy than before, even though my workday was very long and physically arduous. And I found I needed only five hours of sleep a night. I fell asleep quickly and awoke easily—just as George Ohsawa had said in his book. I was the cook and the baker. Every night at home, I prepared the sourdough bread and left it to rise on the heater. Every morning, at a little past five A.M., I baked the bread, prepared the day's food, and transported it to the store. The food was kept warm in double boilers on electric hot plates.

Four changes convinced me of the personal benefits of my macrobiotic practice. First, I began to thoroughly enjoy grains and vegetables—and to feel satisfied by them. Remember that this discovery followed years of my refusing to eat vegetables or anything resembling "real food." My mother had had to strain the vegetables out of my soup before I would consider eating it! Once I began to appreciate vegetables, my incessant craving for junk food faded. The more macrobiotic food I ate, the more I enjoyed it. This was a revelation to someone with a history of always looking for his next snack.

Second, after several months of macrobiotic practice, I noticed that my libido and sexual vitality were increasing. I can't say I'd really noticed a decline, since it had occurred gradually over a period of a few years, but apparently my junk-food diet and abusive lifestyle had weakened me more than I'd realized.

The third change, though, was the most significant. Through macrobiotics, I discovered my direction in life. The future was filled with meaning. Each day was an adventure. I no longer counted the hours until I could go home, as I'd done in every job I'd ever held until then.

And, fourth, I was able, finally, to see the value and power in my own life. When I was growing up, I was full of admiration for nearly everyone else. I believed everyone had better qualities or a better life than I. After practicing macrobiotics for a while, there came a day when I awoke thinking, "I'm glad I'm me." Somehow, I had gained confidence in myself and in my life. I felt refreshed and renewed. I could only attribute this profound change in outlook to my macrobiotic practice and study.

There were just two macrobiotic cookbooks at the time: *Zen Cookery* by George Ohsawa and *Zen Macrobiotic Cooking* by Michel Abehsera. I tried new recipes every day. Cooking became an adventure. I was amazed and excited by how well the dishes turned out. Even non-macrobiotic friends liked them.

The store was my other big adventure. I looked forward to meeting the customers and seeing what they bought and what they ate. Talking with them, and attempting to answer their questions, made me increasingly aware of my own lack of experience and understanding of macrobiotics. My dream was to study with Michio Kushi. Up to this point, my studies had been solely with Rod and Peggy House. Rod had given me my first shiatsu massage and had begun to teach me how to give shiatsu. (Shiatsu, a massage technique that uses finger pressure, has become widely accepted because of its effectiveness in dealing with a variety of common health problems.) Peggy had taught me to cook, and both of them had encouraged me to stay in Philadelphia to develop Essene.

About a month after Essene opened, I visited one of Michio Kushi's study houses in Brookline, Massachusetts. Living in a study house seemed the best way to deepen my understanding of macrobiotics. It would also give me a chance to hear Michio speak. He lectured a few evenings a week, and each lecture was a revelation. To witness his capacity for life, to receive the gift of his understanding of Nature, the universe, health, science, and history was mind altering. I couldn't get enough.

I decided to see Michio for a consultation. He invited me over at lunchtime and didn't stop eating while we talked. After some brief casual conversation, he looked at my palm and told me I was a hard worker. Then he drew the standard macrobiotic diet on a small piece of paper. I asked if I should eat fish. He said, "not much." I asked if there was anything else he had to tell me. He told me to eat miso soup every day. I prodded him some more. He told me about the special leadership seminar he was giving over the summer. I decided then and there to go even though Essene needed my attention.

> "I have never let my schooling interfere with my education."
>
> —Mark Twain

Michio lectured nearly every day for three months during that summer. The topics included macrobiotic philosophy and cooking, shiatsu massage, Oriental diagnosis and medicine, meditation, and other spiritual practices. I felt as if I had finally begun to practice macrobiotics. I had learned so much that was new and inspiring from Michio's lectures and from my stay in the study house. I returned to Philadelphia filled with the spirit of macrobiotics and eager to make Michio's teachings a part of my own life and to share them with others.

About six months after we opened Essene, Stanley disappeared and was never heard from again. So it was that when Rod and Peggy House left for Brookline, I became, by default,

Philadelphia's macrobiotic leader. Although I was only twenty-one at that time, I was the person with the most experience in macrobiotic studies and practice. I began teaching immediately, and within the year I was able to offer private counseling to clients.

Forty-some years have passed since then, and in all that time I have never stopped studying. The focus of my thinking has been and continues to be how best to apply the principles of macrobiotics to the daily strengthening of individual, social, and planetary health.

HOW I DISCOVERED THE STRENGTHENING HEALTH APPROACH

Over the years, I've observed thousands of people practice macrobiotics—some with great success and some with none at all. I've spent a great deal of time trying to pinpoint the difference between a successful practice and a failed one.

Generally speaking, people who undertake the practice of macrobiotics fall into one of two groups: those interested in macrobiotics as a way of life, and those interested in the diet. By and large, those drawn to the macrobiotic philosophy tend to approach macrobiotics with an open mind and a sense of excitement. They don't feel limited or restricted by the practice. On the contrary, they feel they have received the gift of freedom.

Those who come because of the diet, having heard that the diet is strict, limited, and arduous, tend, unfortunately, to model their practice along those lines. Unless the individuals in this group can learn to appreciate macrobiotics as a flexible, harmonious, and satisfying way of life, they often have difficulty adapting to and staying with the practice.

After many years of counseling, I decided it was time to look at how macrobiotics was being presented to the world.

My goal was to find a way to make macrobiotics more open and accessible to the general public. In 1992, in search of insight, my family and I moved to Portugal. We stayed there three years. One beautiful day, while sitting on the beach gazing at the water and enjoying the sunshine, an idea came to me. Why not teach people how and what to *add* to their lives, rather than focus on how and what to give up?

WHAT IS A MACROBIOTIC DIET, ANYWAY?

George Ohsawa introduced macrobiotics to the United States in 1950. He created ten diets that you will find summarized in the following chart. His ten diets ranged from No. 7, a diet consisting only of grains, down to No. −3, a diet consisting of 10% grains and 90% other foods. The numbering is purposeful and the number seven is especially significant. God created the earth in seven days; there are seven days in a week; seven is the number of orbits in a complete spiral.

Diet No.	Grains	Vegetables	Soup	Animal	Salad/Fruit	Dessert
7	100%					
6	90%	10%				
5	80%	20%	10%			
4	70%	30%	10%			
3	60%	30%	10%			
2	50%	30%	10%	10%		
1	40%	30%	10%	20%		
-1	30%	30%	10%	20%	10%	
-2	20%	30%	10%	25%	10%	5%
-3	10%	30%	10%	30%	15%	5%

Doesn't the chart seem to imply that Diet No. 7 is the best one? That Diet No. 6 is not quite as good but still worthy? After all, we marvel at the beauty of six-sided figures like snowflakes or honeycombs. That Diet No. 5 is also appealing, a strong number calling to mind a pentagon? Don't the negative or minus numbers make us feel as if we are being penalized? If this is your thinking, you are not alone. Many people at one time or another have believed that Diet No. 7, in its total devotion to grain, is the ideal.

Although I never met George Ohsawa, Michio and Aveline Kushi believe that his true intention was to show the variety possible in macrobiotic practice and not to rank the diets. Even though Ohsawa was incredibly diverse in his practice and lifestyle, many of those who followed his teachings were not. And many of those who knew Ohsawa personally insist that his teachings alone are valid. He had a kind of power about him that captivated people.

THE KUSHI STANDARD MACROBIOTIC DIET

To dispel the notion that a macrobiotic diet demands adherence to a single plan, the Kushis used another approach. They averaged Ohsawa's ten diets to show the variety and flexibility available in macrobiotic practice. They created the Standard Macrobiotic Diet and made it easily accessible by presenting it as a pie divided into various-sized slices:

- 40% to 60% cereal grains
- 1 to 2 bowls of soup
- 20% to 30% vegetables
- 5% to 10% beans and sea vegetables

- Other foods revolving around the main ones, including condiments, seasonings, nuts, seeds, fruits, sweets, desserts, white-meat fish, and beverages.

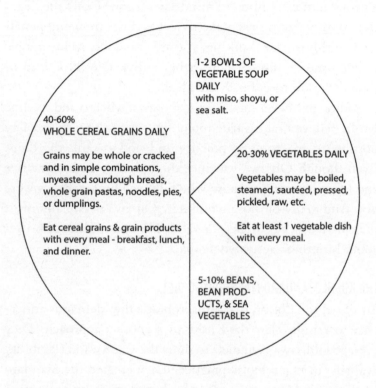

Most people who encounter Ohsawa's standard diet in table form perceive it as rigid, limited, and forbidding. When they see the Kushis' formulation—the pie shape—they envision a plate divided into portions—a visual representation of how a meal should look. Here is the portion of grain, the soup, etc. Here is the macrobiotic way of eating.

Without meaning to, both these approaches somehow give the impression that the goal is a perfect practice. They create the image that macrobiotics is about perfection. But it's always been my belief that the point of macrobiotics is to recreate ourselves each day as who we really want to be. To accomplish this, we must create an orderly life by learning how to make interesting, healthful choices. Perfection, even if there were such a thing, is irrelevant. What we are looking for is an orderly and balanced way of life. Why? Because it is in the nature of things that balance craves more balance.

THE WAXMAN PLAN

The practice of macrobiotics needs to adapt to our changing personal and environmental conditions over time. Through our experience, the higher percentage of grains recommended in the past no longer has the same benefits as they once did. In general, people's conditions have changed due to weaker quality of food and lack of physical activity and contact with the natural environment. Most people spend too much time indoors or sitting at a desk. It's time for a new balance to adapt to modern times.

In our own practice and recommendations, we've been decreasing the percentage of grains and increasing vegetables. We recommend that most people start out with an equal amount of grains and vegetables throughout the day. If your digestion feels heavy, you can try decreasing grains a bit. And if you feel a lack of focus and vitality, you can try increasing grains slightly. We've also found that most people need more beans now than in the past, and we recommend one to one and a half servings of beans/bean products (combinations of beans, tofu, and tempeh) often or daily. A serving of beans is one half to one cup.

Food is our strongest desire. In a contest between a craving and an individual's willpower, the craving always wins. For example, if you consume enough salt, you will feel thirsty and have to drink. If you eat dry toast regularly, sooner or later you will begin to crave something sweet or rich like butter or jam to put on it. If you resist the temptation, you will crave something even sweeter and richer later on. There is no exception. In the end, food always wins. Better to discard the notion that the macrobiotic diet demands perfect obedience. If you don't, trouble will follow.

Our second strongest desire is for sex. Few people can conquer the desire for sex. A strong desire can be suppressed, diminished, or even lost because of declining health, but the loss of desire usually has a harmful effect on the other parts of our lives.

It's easy to extend the idea that if perfection is possible in the areas of diet and sexual activity, it is also possible in other areas of life, in work, for instance, or in relationships. But this is a completely unrealistic concept, and to guide our lives according to it would be supremely foolish and lead only to despair.

According to this kind of wrong-headed thinking, if we should eat something that doesn't fit with our notion of the perfect diet, then we're no longer macrobiotic—the experiment is over. Now let's try a different way of looking at the subject: instead of worrying about giving up certain foods, instead of thinking, "no meat, no chicken, no eggs, no this, no that," why not consider adding foods. Ask yourself "what would be good for me to eat, what would I really like to eat, what will further my life?"

Don't take anything away. Start by adding grains to your present diet. To complement the grains, add vegetables. Follow that by adding soup. Finally, add other foods: beans, sea vegetables, seeds, nuts, fruits, desserts, beverages, and possibly wild, white-meat fish. Where you stop adding is up to you. Do you want to stop with a completely vegan or vegetarian menu, or do you want to include fish? The choice is yours. When you approach the subject this way, the likelihood of your wanting other animal food is remote. In my experience, most people lose their taste for animal and dairy food after they begin eating grains and vegetables. The rewards to mind and body are so enormous that we begin to crave the foods that provide the most benefit and the greatest sense of health and well-being.

As soon as we are told not to have something, it seems we want it all the more. Prohibition increases desire. Whether we really desire it or not is hardly the point. Restriction inevitably leads to excess. Let me give you an example from my own life. I was never much of a fruit eater, but on one particular day in Boston I ate a lot of it. That night, after Michio's lecture, when I went up to ask him a question, he replied only, "Too much fruit." However, in spite of his remark, for the next few weeks I ate more and more fruit. I couldn't stop. It was as if a dam had burst. I don't like fruit all that much and here I was going crazy over it.

Most people find it extremely difficult to give up their favorite foods. We spend our entire lives eating a particular way and even though we may know that the foods we love are making us sick, we cannot give them up without a struggle. Younger people often have a harder time than older ones, perhaps because many older people remember a more natural, orderly way of eating from their own childhood. Our memory for food is very strong and, as we age, our tastes are more likely to revert to the tastes we developed while we were growing up.

The insight I was looking for, the one that came to me that day on the beach in Portugal, was this: Why not begin the practice of macrobiotics by adding healthful foods to the individual's current diet? Why take anything away? Wouldn't this approach help people switch to the macrobiotic diet at their own pace and with less difficulty? My observation since then has been that this approach works pretty well. From that day to this, my dream has been to continue finding new ways to make the practice and value of macrobiotics more open and accessible.

In the mid-eighties, I had developed a program called Discovery that was designed to teach people everything they needed to know about macrobiotics in one day. I also incorporated a very abbreviated version of Discovery into my one-hour counseling sessions. At the time, it was the only way I could think of to help my clients implement the major life-style changes I was recommending to them.

I devoted a five-minute portion of the Discovery program to making the transition to a more healthful diet and lifestyle. I advised people on how to encourage family and friends to change their ways of eating. As a first step, I introduced them to more healthful foods and life-style practices. At the same time, I urged them not to worry about giving up any of the foods they were attached to. But it was not until that day at the beach that I realized just how widely applicable the principle behind Discovery was. In fact, the Discovery program proved to be the seed for this book.

On my regular trips back to the United States during the years I lived in Portugal, I lectured often on the Strengthening Health approach. I offered public seminars and a two-weekend-long course to train people in this approach. When I moved back to the States in 1995, I made a concentrated effort to introduce this approach to as many people as possible. An effort continues to this day at The Strengthening Health Institute, which was founded in 1997 and became a nonprofit in 2002.

Many of the clients who seek my help come to me with serious illnesses, such as cancer and diabetes. Even so, I will sometimes recommend that they add food that is more healthful to their diets before encouraging them to give up the foods they usually eat. With very few exceptions, they gravitate naturally toward the more healthful food.

If we change our diet, even in a limited way, our food cravings change too. Many of us feel guilty or weak-willed if we can't stick to a specific diet. It's important to understand that by eating certain foods, we set ourselves up for failure. Cravings are not a matter of mind control, discipline, or will power but are the expression of a mechanical process. Cravings are a manifestation of the body's desire for balance.

My point is this: if you approach the subject of eating healthfully in a positive manner by thinking of expanding your food choices rather than denying yourself the foods you crave, you are more likely to be successful. Start by selecting grains that satisfy and nourish you. Then choose vegetable dishes and other foods. Make these choices part of your daily meals and, at the same time, make daily exercise a habit. Finally, take a look at the other areas of your life and start to include things that can bring you to balance. After a short while, you will begin to experience a kind of natural satisfaction. Then you can decide how much you want to do on a regular basis in the areas of diet and eating habits, exercise, and lifestyle. The choice is solely yours. Strengthening your health is an ongoing process.

This positive approach is the basic concept underlying Seven Steps to Strengthening Health, and it is a concept that is infinitely adaptable. For instance, you may choose to eat the best organically grown grains and grain products, or you may choose commercial whole wheat or rye bread or pasta as your grain product. This flexibility means that you may practice these principles in a diner, a deli, a fine restaurant, or at home.

The vegetables you select can be of the highest quality, organically grown from your own garden, freshly picked and prepared, or you can order conventionally grown steamed broccoli at an Italian restaurant or at a diner. The same principle applies to soup. The choice runs the gamut from the best homemade organic vegetable soup to jazzed-up canned soup. You may apply these principles across the board—wherever you find yourself. You can adjust food quality up or down, as long as you keep to the format. You may use instant foods, microwave foods, restaurant and takeout foods, or you may choose to prepare the best home-cooked food every day. There are many options and many ways to apply the Strengthening Health principles to your own life. As you can see, what I'm really talking about here is a way of life, an approach to life. What Seven Steps to Strengthening Health offers is an orderly approach to life.

As with most things in life, perception often determines outcome. If you perceive macrobiotics as a closing spiral, one that narrows and limits you, you will most probably abandon it because you will find the practice too difficult and too rigid. If, on the other hand, you conceive of it as an opening spiral, one that expands your freedom and widens your thinking, you will be off on a fabulous lifelong adventure. Your vision and your approach are the catalysts to strengthening your health.

In formulating these ideas, I made a couple of conscious decisions. First, everything I had to say here would derive from collective human experience and wisdom. Second, everything would have a basis in common sense, one of the few qualities of mind I believe in strongly. Scientific theories come and go. Common sense, grounded in human experience, prevails over time. I think it's hard to fault any of the seven steps. I want everyone to be able to prove or disprove these principles through their own experience. I am sure if you try them for two or three weeks, you will see the value they have for your life.

HOW TO USE THIS BOOK

There is something for everyone, and there are multiple points of entry into getting started with *The Complete Macrobiotic Diet*. First, the most important thing is the desire to make changes; everything starts from that point. Since health is a direction, any step in that direction is a benefit. We get benefit from what we do, not from what we don't do. If you're already practicing a vegetarian or vegan diet, you can go to the Healthful Foods List and begin incorporating these foods into your diet. Or you can visit the Recipes section and familiarize yourself with some of the macrobiotic cooking styles. If you're not ready to change your diet, you can look at eating habits or lifestyle practices. You may decide it's time to start walking outside or getting some green plants in your home so they will serve as a reminder of your commitment to your health.

The point is, if we add something healthful into our life, whether or not it's food, we attract other healthful things into our life as well. For most people, a gradual approach is better if there is no need for rapid changes to their health. Progress toward health is like life: some days are better than others. If some days do not go the way you like, try not to let yourself get discouraged. It's a journey, after all, so just try to continue in the direction of health.

The use for a long-time practitioner of macrobiotics is that this book provides an orderly structure to refocus their macrobiotic practice. For those who are new to macrobiotics, my intention was to simplify and rearrange the core of the macrobiotic practice into steps that can be approached systematically. Since balance craves balance, anything that is balanced in your life will move you in the direction of health. I think it is better to practice at your own pace and to introduce each new step once you are ready than to bite off more than you can chew and become overwhelmed. It's easier to give up once you become overwhelmed. Some of my clients don't come back, or give up, because they feel like they cannot practice according to my recommendations. Again, it's not about being perfect, but creating health supporting habits over time.

This book is also intended to be a handbook to guide you toward health. The steps are simplified, yet also condensed. As your practice advances and evolves, each time you visit this book, you may find something new to think about or add to your practice.

Another important use of this book is to share this understanding with others. I hope it will be the beginning of many good conversations. I also hope you will make these principles a part of your life in the spirit of joy and adventure. Allow common sense to guide you. Observe the benefits that come from your practice. Should you find you are not getting the desired results, adjust what you are doing. Talk to those who have more experience and who can guide you. Try to proceed in the spirit of the early explorers who left the old ways behind in their search for greater freedom and richer lives. If you can do this, you will discover a quality of health that is life-changing. Please use it well and share it with others.

Spread the joy, spread the health!

CONNECTING WITH
THE SPIRIT OF HEALTH

"We are one with Nature and the environment."
—a rough translation of *Shindo Fuji*,
which George Ohsawa used to
formulate the macrobiotic
philosophy and lifestyle

GIVING THANKS FOR OUR FOOD
"The noblest question in the world is What
Good may I do in it?"
—Benjamin Franklin

The orderly cycles of Nature guide this book and my macrobiotic practice. Through aligning with these orderly cycles, we
reconnect with all aspects of Nature. For life on this planet,
we observe this orderliness through days, seasons, years, and
growth cycles. Food is our connection to Nature. When
eating plants directly from Nature, we create a direct connection, which fosters a care and love of self and planet. When

we eat plants that have already been processed by animals, we create an indirect connection.

All food has three types of nourishment: physical, energetic, and spiritual.

Physical nourishment is the basic constituent of food, the raw material that we digest and process. Physical nourishment gives us energy and becomes our blood, tissues, and organs. The principal categories of physical nourishment are minerals, proteins, carbohydrates, fats, vitamins, and enzymes.

Energetic nourishment is the nourishment we derive from the food as a result of its life cycle—from growth to our plates. For plants, energetic nourishment begins with the quality of both the seed and the soil within which they grow. The process continues and includes the harvest, how the plants grow, how we process, store, distribute and finally, prepare them for consumption. Energetic nourishment is the food quality.

Modern agriculture has lost touch with the common sense of our ancestral agriculture. We have a worldwide history of small, local farms producing nourishing food on a community basis. There is a clear connection between healthy soil, healthy plants, and healthy people. How can we expect to have healthy people without healthy food?

Spiritual nourishment is the nourishment derived from the health and intention of the person or people preparing the food. Our care and love transforms the physical and energetic properties of the food into the most nourishing food. This type of food gives us the most satisfaction and inspires in us a profound sense of gratitude. Everyone knows how wonderful holiday meals are and the way they can stand out in our memory.

Food is our life. Without food, there is no life. When we start with food that is naturally grown and processed and prepared with care and love, we have something that is unfortunately rare and unique in today's society. Food prepared with care and love, even without using the highest quality ingredients, is still satisfying and nourishing. Most people will agree that the spiritual aspect of nourishment is the most satisfying, followed by energetic. The energetic aspect is enhanced when the food grows naturally and origi nates close to where we live. Food from your garden always tastes the best.

> "When eating fruit, remember who planted the tree; when drinking water, remember who dug the well."
>
> —Vietnamese Proverb

Giving thanks before and after a meal literally wakes up the goodness in the food. We become aware by appreciating and acknowledging the entire process of our food. We give thanks for the whole network that connects us to that food, which in turn allows us to be nourished and satisfied at a much deeper level. Our gratitude for food opens us to health, to life and all of its possibilities.

HEALTH CRAVES HEALTH

> "Preserve and treat your food as you would your body, remembering that in time food will be your body."
>
> —B. W. Richardson

Health is natural. Our bodies want to be healthy; it is really our default state. We know this because if we develop a serious health problem, it takes far less time to return to health than it did to become sick in the first place. It often takes many years to spoil our health, yet most people could turn their health around in six months to a year. If we allow it, our body is always trying to maintain or return to health. Most people think that being healthy seems to require a lot of discipline. The focus is on taking away rather than adding.

My experience is the opposite. Adding is more important than taking away. Giving things up does not lead to lasting health. When I started to add healthful foods to my diet, I realized that I had started to crave more foods that supported my health all of the time. It became apparent that it wasn't only food. My desires started to extend to other areas of life. At the same time, I started to lose interest in things that weren't supportive of my health and life. I believe this pattern is common for everyone. The opposite is also true. Once we start to eat unhealthful foods, we surround ourselves with more destructive food, habits, and tendencies. This is why fast foods and junk foods have been able to take over so strongly.

Health is simple. I find it interesting that many people think that health is not attainable for two main reasons. One, people think that becoming healthy requires too much effort. The second main reason is they think that genetic and/or environmental factors undermine our daily efforts. It is easy to assume that sickness is inevitable no matter what we do. It has recently been discovered that there are factors that have more influence than genetics alone. Epigenetics offers scientific support that daily choices are responsible for the activation and expression of genes that regulate the disease process, including cancer genes. Diet and lifestyle factors have the ability to turn gene markers on or off. In my experience, daily things, not special things, create health. Good food, natural activity, and a healthy attitude are the most important factors to create lasting health.

Health craves health. We start with good eating habits. Then we add healthful foods and cooking styles into our way of eating. We further the process with natural activities and try to create a healthy home environment. These things work together to move us in the direction of health. This process becomes self-sustaining: that is, it does not require discipline.

> "What we are doing to the forests of the world is but a mirror reflection of what we are doing to ourselves and to one another."
> —Mahatma Gandhi

Personal health and planetary health are the same. Healthy people want to live in a healthy home environment, and the desire extends to a healthy, natural environment. As we take better care of our own health, all of our choices begin to support our community and environment. As we become more calm, more peaceful, and more positive, we begin to spread these things around us. When we eat naturally grown and processed foods, we don't spoil the environment. When we eat grains and beans directly, as opposed to feeding them to animals, we make enough food available for everyone. We are also, in turn, naturally much kinder to animals. We also no longer need to clear-cut forests to raise animals. The desire to seek health is an open-ended cycle.

Health is contagious. Healthy people naturally want to support Community-supported agriculture organizations (CSAs), farmer's markets, and other practices that support a healthier environment; it is not a matter of discipline, but desire. The proliferation of CSAs, farmer's markets, seed exchanges, and artisanal food products reflects the growing number of people who are experiencing the life-changing effects of craving health.

LASTING HEALTH, A SPIRITUAL QUALITY

Illness surrounds us; heart disease, cancer, dementia, and diabetes have reached epidemic levels. From this, it is natural to assume that we are likely to die from at least one degenerative illness. However, there are cultures and communities around the world whose older members are just as vital and bright as those much younger. Take Okinawa, where they have the highest life expectancy. Their diet and lifestyle practices produce more centenarians than anywhere else in the world. Many people there have been able to delay, or even avoid, the "diseases of aging."

"The belly rules the mind."

—Spanish Proverb

George Ohsawa, the founding father of modern-day macrobiotics, created a unique definition of health. Michio Kushi further refined, adapted, and developed his definition. They divided health into three main areas: physical, mental/ emotional, and spiritual health. Conditions of physical health are a strong physical and mental vitality, a good appetite for healthy food, and deep and refreshing sleep. You can achieve five points for each condition. Ideal physical health amounts to fifteen points. Mental/emotional conditions of health include good memory, being calm and patient, and being joyous and alert. Mental/emotional conditions of health receive ten points and amount to thirty in total. The condition of spiritual health is the endless appreciation for all of life, and the spiritual total is 55 points. You need this condition to be a healthy person, as it accounts for more than half of all the points. This definition is unique because it shows that we have the ability to grow and create our health throughout our life. This point system allows us to check our health on a regular basis, but it is most important on a seasonal or yearly basis.

Macrobiotics is a lifestyle through which we can grow spiritually and also develop our mental, emotional, and physical health, which allows us to lead the most exciting and fulfilling life. Lasting health is our ability to grow and nourish our health on all levels throughout our life. There is no limit to our vitality, memory, sense of joy, or appreciation of life.

Gratitude and appreciation open us to life and all of its possibilities. Even if we are not raised with a deep sense of appreciation and gratitude, we still have the ability to achieve this spiritual quality. Life's challenges offer us the opportunity to develop this appreciation. It is my long observation that people with a deep appreciation have the greatest ability to overcome life's challenges. Many of my clients have attributed their recovery to their sense of appreciation of life.

INDIGENOUS & LOCAL FOODS
Indigenous Food: The Soil Principle
Indigenous foods are foods that are native to a growing region; they have evolved and adapted over long periods of

time to particular, unique climates and ecosystems. Food grows in perfect balance with local conditions, in accordance with soil and water quality, temperature, humidity, patterns of sunlight, etc. To eat indigenous food is to eat foods that have adapted to the locality. Where a food was originally cultivated in relation to our own regions matters far more than whether or not the food is local.

When we eat food that is native or climatically similar to our own region, it is easier to digest, absorb its nutrition, and eliminate excess. Indigenous foods align us to our locality so we can connect more easily to what we eat and the natural conditions where we live. When we eat foods that are native to our climatic region, the food harmonizes our metabolism to that region. The pace of life is more active in the temperate climatic regions than in the tropics and sub-tropics. When we eat food from the tropics and sub-tropics in a temperate zone, the food regulates our metabolism to the tropics and we disconnect from the natural pace of our own environment.

From my experience, foods from sub-tropical and tropical climates introduced to a temperate-climatic diet cause the blood to become more acidic than any other plant-based foods. We lose minerals and other nutrients trying to neutralize the acidity. When we have acidic conditions, we become more susceptible to infectious, inflammatory, and degenerative illnesses. When our blood is more acidic, the hemoglobin loses its ability to bind with and transport oxygen throughout our body. Our ability to absorb nutrients also becomes compromised. Two types of foods that evolved in the tropics and sub-tropics are the thick-skinned tropical fruits and the nightshades.

I find it very interesting that five tropical foods have become so deeply ingrained in our diet, even though they all negatively affect our health: potatoes, tomatoes, sugar, bananas, and, more recently, coconuts. They are all tropical and highly acidifying to our blood. We know that nightshades have a strongly acidifying effect. Those with arthritis are usually affected by eating these foods. The perception of these foods as healthful in a temperate region does not consider the role that local and indigenous foods play with our health.

From my observation, people with a healthy metabolism never have to think about their weight. Many of my clients who come for a variety of health problems naturally lose weight as they improve their health in other areas. When the body begins to function naturally again, it actively releases toxins and other forms of excess. Could it be that all these tropical foods are interfering with our ability to eliminate excess, as well as exacerbating the obesity epidemic?

An indigenous food can be considered indigenous along a line of latitude, not longitude. Which means we can choose foods east and west of where we live around the world. For example, cherry blossoms are enjoyed in both Washington, D.C. and Kyoto, Japan. For those in the temperate climatic regions, there is not as much flexibility in choosing foods north and south as the climate changes dramatically. It is best to choose foods within the temperate zones rather than the sub-tropics or tropics.

The problem, though, is not the banana or the coconut, it is the proportions of consumption of tropical fruits and nightshades in relation to the indigenous foods we eat. It is best to use these foods with care and discretion. If you are unsure about which foods are indigenous to temperate climatic zones, you can consult the food list in the back of this book.

Since food is our direct connection to the entire network of life, indigenous and local foods in combination are the foods that are most healthful for us, as they are best adapted to where we live.

Local Food: The Water Principle

The local food movement gains momentum day to day, week to week, farmers' market to farmers' market, season to season. Getting our food and exchanging with local growers increases our awareness of the life cycles of our food. It also gives us the opportunity to experience the changing seasons and connect with what grows in our area. We look forward to the first strawberry of mid-spring and for the first peach of the summer. We somehow understand that foods grown locally make more sense for the overall planet and ourselves, but apart from reducing our dependence on fossil fuels, local foods also help us to align with the rhythms of Nature.

Food becomes unique to a locality. The food grown in a specific area experiences the changes and patterns according to the conditions and quality of the weather, the water, the soil, and many other factors. Food local to our area has essentially had a similar experience to ours, except that food metabolizes the environment directly. We can feel this connection through our experience with spring fever. In plants, energy rises, sap begins to run, buds form, and we become excited to be out and experience the warmth and witness Nature coming back to life. When we eat local foods, we connect to the experience of the season and can receive better nourishment. Food absorbs minerals directly from the soil, and local foods allow us to absorb these minerals more efficiently.

Water is the most important thing to have locally, as it quickly loses its freshness. Water from a spring does not taste the same, once we take it home, as it does while at the spring! Most leafy vegetables have a high water content; the higher the water content in a vegetable, the more important it becomes for the vegetable to be from a local source. Vegetables with high water content lose their nutritive value and freshness faster than vegetables that can be stored for a longer period of time. However, vegetables grown locally on good soil also store water better than others. If we get the vegetables locally, we maximize the nutritional benefit from the growth and harvest process as well as take in the available water in the plant.

The most important source of water is in food. We use water in food more efficiently than by just drinking alone. If we contrast this with the modern diet, we can see that almost all of the foods in the modern diet are dry foods, such as meat, poultry, cheese, eggs, and baked goods. These foods create an imbalance of thirst. People have perpetual thirst, but don't seem satisfied, whereas eating food that has a high moisture content satisfies our need for liquids more deeply. All cooked grains, beans, pastas, vegetables, and soups have high water content. The taste of these foods becomes sweeter and more thirst-quenching as we chew them. These healthful foods allow us to become more satisfied with drinks and beverages that we choose to enjoy. The water in food refreshes us, and we cherish foods that are considered refreshing (ex.: lettuce, cucumbers, and of course watermelon). Refreshing is a vital nutrient.

Locality is less important to consider for vegetables that can be stored. Storing vegetables (cabbages, onions, carrots, sweet potatoes, hard fruits, etc.) used to carry people through barren winters. Harder vegetables have more adaptability, that is, they can store in a variety of environments without rapidly decaying. Fruits that can be stored, such as apples and pears, become more nutritious and better tasting during cold storage as the flavors settle down and concentrate.

Grains, beans, dried vegetables, and seaweeds store for much longer than other foods. Therefore, these foods can come from farther away, even anywhere in the country, or from the same hemisphere. Foods from opposite sides of the equator have an opposite magnetic charge and should be avoided. These foods interfere with our body's functions as well as our connection to our locality. Finally, we cook our food using local, filtered water, which completes the cycle. You can start to make a more local transition by using water content as the guide. Visit farmers' markets to first get leafy vegetables and local, seasonal fruits, and follow this with more substantial vegetables. Enjoy your way through the seasons as they change.

> "Here is your country. Cherish these natural wonders, cherish the natural resources, cherish the history and the romance as a sacred heritage, for your children and your children's children. Do not let selfish men or greedy interests skin your country of its beauty, its riches or its romance."
>
> —Theodore Roosevelt

As we start to choose more indigenous and local foods, we start to make a deeper and more satisfying connection to where we live. This enhances our ability to make healthful choices for our own lives. We start to create a balance through indigenous and local foods that also helps us to become more deeply satisfied from the foods we do eat. This balance continues to perpetuate itself. The reality is that the most healthful food is the most enjoyable food.

ACID & ALKALINE, OVEREATING, AND GLUTEN SENSITIVITY: A MACROBIOTIC PERSPECTIVE

ACID AND ALKALINE

I found it necessary to reinterpret acid and alkaline to make it more effective and easier to understand. I am not a scientist, but this interpretation is based on my understanding of macrobiotics. This understanding has passed the test of time, as I've used it with clients over the years to create healthy, alkaline conditions. People have said that grains and beans are acidifying, but that has not been my experience. I think you'll find when grains and beans are cooked in water with a little sea salt or kombu, and digested properly, they create alkaline conditions. If this wasn't so, macrobiotics would not have such a large number of recoveries from serious illnesses, which is what it is so well known for. My observation throughout the years is that macrobiotic children have been stronger and healthier than their peers not raised in this way. Healthy digestion, which starts with thorough chewing, is essential for creating a mildly alkaline condition.

When digested properly, complex carbohydrates, such as grains and beans, and temperate land and sea vegetables create a mildly alkaline condition in the blood. On the other hand, simple sugars, refined carbohydrates, and alcohol quickly become absorbed into the bloodstream, creating an acidic condition. Animal and dairy foods, tropical fruits, and nightshades also acidify the blood. We lose minerals, especially calcium, to neutralize the acidity. This loss of minerals weakens not only our bones, but our muscles, organs, and nervous system. It also weakens our digestive and thinking abilities.

For food to become alkalized, three important things must happen. First, we need to sit down to eat without doing other things. Second, food must be chewed well. The third is that complex carbohydrates must slowly break down in the digestive process, alkalize in the duodenum, and finally be absorbed in the small intestine. A combination of complex carbohydrates creates the most healthy alkaline condition. In essence, the importance is to differentiate between good-quality and poor-quality carbohydrates because the complex carbohydrates are the ones that break down slowly and pass through the duodenum.

Create alkalinity with food by eating a variety of complex carbohydrates that are digested slowly, and are absorbed in the small intestine. In life, anything that promotes good digestion and circulation promotes alkalinity: chewing our food, laughter, a nice walk outside, a great conversation, green plants, natural materials and activity, etc. Alkaline conditions allow hemoglobin to bind with more oxygen and transport it through our body. Indicators of an alkaline condition include a sense of inner peace and joy, having a positive attitude, feeling strong and energetic, good muscle tone, healthy skin, and youthful appearance.

Acidic conditions are caused by stagnation. Overeating is one of the most common causes of stagnation and acidity in our body. Contrast the freshness of a walk outside with one in a shopping mall or sitting in front of a computer all day. Common symptoms of acidity are fatigue, negativity, irritability, weak bones and muscles, and a weak resistance to illness.

You can get a pretty decent indicator of your overall condition by observing how you wake up and feel every day.

OVEREATING

Overeating is one of the most harmful and common habits that many people experience today. Eating while standing or doing other things sets the stage. The most common practices that break our connection with food are reading, watching TV, or listening to engaging radio broadcasts while trying to eat. These practices interfere with our digestion and feelings of satisfaction. Another cause for overeating is having a diet that is too simple and repetitive where we try to get satisfaction by eating more and more food. Eating unhealthful foods causes a biological frustration and imbalance that causes us to overeat. One unhealthful food makes you crave another.

My analogy is this: If you have a comfortable number of people in a room, people tend to be thoughtful and accommodating to everyone else. However, if you double the number of people in the room beyond the capacity of the room, the same caring people often become irritable and negative instead. The same goes for the food we eat. Once we eat beyond our capacity, we start to bring out the negative aspects of the food.

There is a physical limitation as to how much our digestive system can process and eliminate. Overeating can cause food to putrefy in our digestive system and creates the buildup of toxins. This also produces a more acidic condition, as the food cannot move naturally and efficiently through our digestive system.

Another analogy is the mountain stream. As long as the stream can move and flow naturally, it continually cleans and purifies itself. However, if a boulder falls and breaks the natural movement of the stream, stagnation builds up around the boulder. Overeating creates stagnation which interferes with the natural movement of the digestive system. Overeating healthful food is harmful enough, and overeating unhealthful foods brings out the worst aspects of the worst foods.

Almost everyone overeats these days, and it may be difficult for you to tell if you are overeating. A good rule of thumb that they say in Okinawa is to "only eat to 80% capacity." If you're not sure what that feels like, try reducing the overall volume of food by 5-10% at each meal. Then try it again until you get down to a comfortable amount. Once you get used to this, you'll feel more energetic and clear-headed.

GLUTEN ALLERGIES AND SENSITIVITY

Grains are currently under attack as a cause of many modern Western illnesses. The two most widely consumed grains in the world are rice and wheat. Attacks on rice are for arsenic contamination and phytic acid's role in mineral absorption.

Attacks on wheat are for its gluten content and for being over-hybridized. The following is based on my understanding of diet and health and my experience with my students and clients over time. I have helped many people overcome their gluten sensitivities completely.

The common grains containing gluten are wheat, barley, and rye. These grains are amongst the most ancient grains, and wheat in particular has been cultivated as early as 16,000 B.C. in Egypt. All long-standing civilizations and their cuisines developed and evolved using grains as a primary source of nourishment. For more information about what a grain actually is, I provide an overview in Step 3.

Whole grains provide the ideal balance between minerals, proteins, and carbohydrates, making them the most complete source of nutrition of any food. Gluten is a combination of two proteins and is found in the endosperm (or starchy part) of certain cereal grains and gives dough its texture. Grains essentially have encapsulated within them the entire life cycle from seed to fruit, so they are the vital food that provides and maintains the foundation of our nutrition.

There are three parts to the problem with the modern treatment of grains. First, it is true that many modern grains have become over-hybridized, sacrificing quality for yield. In addition, modern milling practices disturb the quality of the grain. Modern milling employs the use of steel hammers, which develop excessive heat. Slow-grinding stone mills preserve the quality of the grain because of the gentle grind. Thirdly, refining and enriching the grain disturbs the nutritional balance. This works like shattering a mirror and merely pasting it together and expecting it to look and function the same as before. Although enriched and refined grains have the same amount of nutrients as a whole grain, they are nutrients out of context with where they came from and do not act the way the nutrients do in whole grains. It is likely that the combination of modern grain and our overall weakened health caused by imbalanced diet and lifestyle are the causes of gluten sensitivity, which is more like an allergic reaction. It's also important to differentiate between gluten allergy/sensitivity and celiac disease. These guidelines are not for people with celiac disease, who should avoid gluten completely.

The science of epigenetics demonstrates that diet and lifestyle regulate the way genes express themselves, which means that autoimmune diseases may reverse themselves over time with healthful diet and lifestyle practices. Many people have reported recovery from degenerative illnesses through dietary and lifestyle changes. A healthy person has the capacity to enjoy Nature and life at its fullest, which includes the complete enjoyment of the foods eaten for thousands of years by the world's long-standing civilizations. Food and environmental allergies have become rampant in our society. Allergies are results and indicators of imbalances, and are related to a weakened blood, lymph, and digestive quality, caused mostly by an overly rich or nutritionally imbalanced diet. Gluten sensitivity is an allergy of the digestive system. The base cause of digestive issues is the overconsumption of strong animal foods, especially red meat, poultry, eggs, and cheese. Our digestive system is not designed to primarily digest and process animal foods efficiently.

Dairy foods confuse our immune system, and sugar paralyzes its ability to react appropriately. The immune system filters our blood and neutralizes acidity. Excessive consumption of dairy foods and poor-quality fats clogs and stagnates our immune system. They interfere with its ability to filter blood. In essence, the function of the immune system is to gather, localize, and neutralize toxins. The immune system does not fight—it harmonizes and balances. The highly expansive nature of simple sugars (such as white sugar and fructose) incapacitates our immune system's ability to gather and localize toxins when consumed above a certain level. Only the liver can metabolize fructose, whereas all the cells in our body metabolize glucose. The combination of dairy foods and fructose especially affects the liver, the spleen, the pancreas, and the immune system in general. In Oriental medicine, the liver and gallbladder are nourished and balanced specifically from the grains containing gluten. In a diet too highly saturated with dairy foods and fructose (especially high-fructose corn syrup and agave nectar), our liver and immune-system functions are compromised and may react inappropriately to these grains.

Two things cause allergic symptoms: the cause of the problem, and what relieves the problem. In other words, symptoms cannot tell us directly whether a problem is getting better or worse. My experience also shows that people produce symptoms when they are recovering their health, which makes the healing process seem scary to many. We've associated symptoms with illness itself, which is not the case.

There is a huge difference between boiled grains such as brown rice or bulgur wheat and baked or toasted grain products. Baked, toasted, fried, yeasted, refined, and enriched grains (such as donuts, cookies, pastries, and commercial breakfast cereals, to name a few) seem to cause the worst reactions. From my experience, many people who are gluten-sensitive are not affected by wheat or barley cooked or boiled together with brown rice. If people react to wheat or barley cooked with brown rice, it is a barometer that usually indicates that there is a more serious issue that requires more time to recover from.

Our body is meant to run on the complex carbohydrates especially found in whole grains, beans, vegetables, seaweeds, and other unrefined, plant-based foods. These foods go through the entire digestive process and are eventually absorbed by the small intestine. Simple carbohydrates (such as enriched and refined grain) become absorbed directly into the blood before they go through the duodenum where they would otherwise naturally go through an alkalizing process. Baking or toasting these refined grains using dry heat can convert complex carbohydrates into trisaccharides, which also causes them to be absorbed by the blood more quickly and may spike the blood sugar.

Baking and toasting are important cooking methods, and I am in no way suggesting that we stop enjoying them. However, their overuse with many refined foods and added sugars contributes to the imbalances in our health. Boiling the grain aids in our ability to efficiently digest and absorb its nutrition.

For those with gluten sensitivity, there are methods to try to reintroduce grain. First, avoid the foods with gluten that you know cause you to experience a reaction. Then, slowly and systematically reintroduce barley, farro, or wheat cooked with brown rice. Then, one by one, reintroduce other boiled, unrefined grains. If they cause a reaction, wait at least ten days and then try again. Then when you're ready, try to introduce soup seasoned with naturally fermented miso. If you have difficulty or continue to experience reactions, you may want to consult with an experienced macrobiotic counselor.

There is a lot of confusion about soy products as well. My experience is that the traditional soy products, which include miso, natural soy sauce, tofu, and tempeh are all protective against estrogen-related illness. It's been found in China and Japan that traditional soy products are protective against breast cancer. In addition, these traditional soy products have a rich array of nutrition and are helpful in practicing a healthful vegan diet.

I hope you will not be dissuaded from eating foods that have been enjoyed by people for thousands of years that provide wonderful health benefits, taste delicious, and even give us emotional satisfaction and fulfillment.

THE
7 STEPS

The Strengthening Health Method proposes an orderly approach to eating and living. It is based on creating healthful eating habits, a balanced diet, and beneficial lifestyle practices. With this in mind, let's get started on the 7 Steps.

"Health, without which there is no happiness."
— Thomas Jefferson

EATING HABITS: FORMAT OF MEALS

1. Take time for your meals everyday.
   - Sit down to eat your meals or snacks without reading, watching TV, or working.
   - Allow adequate time for your meals.
   - Eat slowly and chew well.
   - Stop eating 3 hours before bedtime.
   - Eat in an orderly manner.
   - Avoid mixing foods in the same mouthful.

2. Set your daily schedule.
   - Rise early and go to sleep before midnight.
   - Keep your mealtimes regular.

DIET: CONTENT AND QUALITY OF MEALS
3. Eat 2 or 3 complete and nutritionally balanced meals every day.
- Plan every meal around cooked grains and grain products.
- Complete and balance every meal with 1 or 2 vegetable dishes.
- Have a serving of soup with one of your meals.
- Buy the highest quality organically grown, unrefined, naturally processed and non-GMO foods.

LIFESTYLE: APPROACH TO HEALTH
4. Make your daily life active.
- Walk outside for at least 30 minutes every day.
- Give yourself a daily body rub.
- Life-related exercise provides the most benefit for lasting health.
- Cultivate and take time for hobbies.

5. Create a more natural environment.
- Surround yourself with green plants, especially in the bedroom, the kitchen, the bathrooms, and office or workspace.
- Wear pure cotton clothing next to your skin.
- Use natural materials such as wood, cotton, silk, and wool in your home.

6. Make your macrobiotic practice work.
- Keeping to the format of meals improves your ability to make healthful food choices.

- Keep a daily record of your meals to help you become more objective about your practice.

7. Cultivate the spirit of health.
   - Be open, curious, and endlessly appreciative of all of life.
   - Be flexible and adaptable in your practice.
   - Develop a strong will and the determination to create your own health.
   - Be accurate in your practice.
   - Create a good support network.
   - Learn to cook well.

"Ill-health, of body or of mind, is defeat. Health alone is victory. Let all men, if they can manage it, contrive to be healthy."

—Thomas Carlyle

THE ORIGIN OF THE 7 STEPS

Where do the 7 Steps come from? In other words, what is the model on which they are based? The answer is simple. They are based on my observation of Nature. If we observe Nature closely over time, two clear patterns emerge. The first is that Nature is orderly and consistent. As a result, its cycles are 100% predictable. For example, we know that the sun will rise and set every day. We know the exact time at which this will happen. We know the exact position the sun will occupy in the sky at any given moment. We can predict where it will be at any time in the future. We can project backwards with the same certainty. The sun never takes a break, never takes a day off. If the sun fails to rise, either there is no more sun or our planet is out of orbit. Either way, our worries will be over! We also know that every month, without exception, the moon will move from new to full and back again, as surely as we know that every year, spring will follow winter and summer will follow spring. However, we can never be certain what any individual season, month, week, day, or hour will be like. Sometimes May is atypically rainy and cold while June can be as hot as August. From this observation we can conclude that Nature is orderly and consistent while at the same time it is endlessly variable and inconsistent. These are Nature's two patterns. Simple, yet it seems that in the practice of macrobiotics the two most difficult concepts to understand are those of balance and variety.

> "Common sense and nature will do a lot to make the pilgrimage of life not too difficult."
> —W. Somerset Maugham

BALANCE

If, as I am proposing, our sense of balance comes directly from Nature, then the easiest way to achieve balance is to align with Nature's orderly cycles. To choose to align with endless variety, inconsistency, and change is obviously to choose failure. But we can easily align with the very orderly aspects of Nature—its cycles of sunrise, sunset, and seasons.

VARIETY

Let's take a look at the principle of variety as it applies to macrobiotics. In macrobiotics we believe that everything has its complementary opposite, some other aspect that completes it or brings it to wholeness or to oneness: day—night, man—woman, heat—cold, happiness—sadness, health—sickness, etc. This is true for Nature as well. Its orderly cycles are complemented and completed by its cycles of endless variety, change, and inconsistency. These are Nature's two aspects, or you might say Nature's front and back. The point is that the way we can best align with Nature's variety is through Nature's orderly cycles. This is key to our understanding.

APPETITE

With this in mind, I'd like to pose another basic question. Where does our appetite come from? What determines what our appetite is on any given day, month, or year? Many years ago, when there were a number of macrobiotic study houses in Philadelphia and the community was very closely knit, on any given day you could be sure that almost exactly the same meal was being served in all the different locations—dish for dish, sometimes ingredient for ingredient. Why? We could, I suppose, blame it on gossip. The macrobiotic grapevine is amazingly efficient! However, these different study houses were not sharing menu plans. There is a principle at work behind the similarity, and it is that the nature of each day calls for certain types of food, certain dishes. And so the people who were more aligned with Nature were all drawn to the same foods. In other words, their appetites were aligned with Nature and therefore with each other, so that when they planned their meals they chose nearly identical foods and cooking styles.

Our appetite, our taste, and sense of variety all come from Nature. Now let me take this a step further. Some people argue that having a set schedule is too rigid a way to live. But if we look at Nature, it's hard to say that Nature is rigid. Nature is full of change and inconsistency. Nature is asymmetrical and Nature has no lack of vitality. If you cut things down, they will grow again. Whatever we do to the earth, the earth has the ability to adjust, adapt, repair, and maintain itself. Based on this observation, we can say that Nature has great vitality.

> "After you have exhausted what there is in business, politics, conviviality, and so on—have found that none of these finally satisfy, or permanently wear— what remains? Nature remains."
>
> —Walt Whitman

VITALITY

Where does this vitality come from? I have an answer that satisfies me. You might agree with it, you might not. I believe Nature's vitality is the result of its orderliness. For example, if you grow up in an orderly family, one that has structure, routines, and traditions, one that values consistency so that you know what to expect, then automatically you have a kind of confidence and a vitality for life. Whereas if you grow up in a family where nothing is consistent and life is disorderly, you don't have that positive kind of vitality. Let's suppose, for the purpose of argument, that you have job security and that you know what's expected of you. In such a situation, you can work hard and efficiently without becoming exhausted. But if your job is in jeopardy from day to day and you're not sure what is expected of you, exhaustion sets in almost automatically. Am I right? You lose your energy. You lose your vitality. You lose your creativity. Can you see the influence order and structure exert over our lives and health? Order and structure are what give us vitality, adaptability and creativity, confidence and a zest for life.

If you talk with very old people about their lives, you will discover that what most of them have in common is an orderly life. Set times for sleeping, waking, and meals, times that don't vary. These people are self-sufficient. They rarely, if ever, see doctors. They prefer to guide their own lives and to take care of all their needs themselves. Generally, they live simply. And, because over the years they have maintained this orderliness, they have been rewarded with good health, strong vitality, and long life.

STRUCTURE AND CREATIVITY

I read about an experiment that was done some time ago that is pertinent to what we're talking about. The researchers asked a certain number of people who had had no previous experience in the field of advertising to come up with slogans for various products. The subjects were offered no guidelines whatsoever. The same thing was asked of computers, but since computers can't function without being programmed, the computers were given very clear guidelines. The results didn't surprise me, although they may have surprised the researchers. The slogans the human subjects came up with were too boring and childish to attract any attention. The computers, on the other hand, produced highly creative material that was as good as any dreamt up by the world's most successful advertising agencies. The difference from the macrobiotic point of view was that the human subjects were given no guidelines, no structure, while the computers were given explicit instructions—this is what we want, this is what you may do, this is what you may not do. The point is that alignment with Nature's orderly cycles is the key to understanding variety. It is the key that unlocks freshness and creativity.

SEVEN STEPS

Some of you may have seen the 7 Steps bookmark, all seven steps printed on a slender bookmark. When I lecture, I often say to people that now they know everything I know. People think I'm joking, but I'm not. I'm very serious. If you do these things and bring yourself into alignment with Nature, then you and I will be receiving life from the same source—including our appetite, food choices, ideas, and understanding. We all have the ability to align with Nature and its orderly cycles. All we need is the will and to be shown the way.

I hope that now you can appreciate why an explanation of Eating Habits: Format of Meals had to precede an exploration of the actual Diet: Content of Meals. Eating Habits are the controlling factor. The bottom line is that good eating habits create the ability to make healthful choices. Let's say I fill a table with the best quality and most delicious macrobiotic food and you eat nothing but food from that table. Will that be a guarantee of good health? I don't think so. You won't achieve good health until you learn how to choose the foods you need. We build our health one day at a time, one meal at a time. You must learn to choose appropriately.

The question is, of course, how do we do this? Again, the answer is by adhering to a structure, by incorporating the structure of the 7 Steps into our daily lives.

EATING HABITS: FORMAT OF MEALS

STEP 1

TAKE TIME FOR YOUR MEALS EVERY DAY

Sit down to eat your meals or snacks without reading, watching TV, or working.

> "One of the very nicest things about life is the way we must regularly stop whatever it is we are doing and devote our attention to eating."
> —Luciano Pavarotti

This is the first step toward good health and will help you feel more satisfied. Sitting down to eat is an expression of our appreciation and respect for our food. Sitting down enables us to create order in our daily eating habits and it makes us more conscious of what we eat. The tendency is not to count the food we eat while standing. It just doesn't enter our consciousness. In fact, we usually stand when eating the foods we really don't want to eat or shouldn't be eating. If you tend to snack throughout the day, you will have trouble regulating your meals and perhaps have some difficulty with weight control. Generally, we don't realize how much food we ingest when we are eating constantly. Remember that many people eat not because they are hungry but out of a desire to soothe their nerves or lessen their frustration. For them, food acts as a tranquilizer. If this is true in your case, you will become more aware of it if you sit down whenever you snack. You may even decide you don't really want to eat at that time.

Chinese medicine says that food has both physical aspects and *chi* (or energetic) aspects. If you want to absorb the energetic aspects of your food, your stomach must be in the bent position it takes when you are seated, not in the elongated position it assumes when you stand. As I see it, different positions are for different activities. Standing is for being active and productive; reclining, which is a receptive position, is for sleep, sex, and rest; and sitting is a transitional position between the two postures. We eat during the day so that we have the energy to be active. We sleep at night so that the body, using the food consumed during the day, can repair and maintain itself.

SITTING, STANDING, AND LYING DOWN
Sitting is the link between standing and lying down. Think about how the seated position aligns with eating. The seated position is the one in which the change between the external and internal environments, between giving out and taking in, occurs. Sitting is the position for receiving nourishment, for strengthening the ability to absorb, digest, and assimilate food. It is also the position most congenial to the process of

thinking. Try reading while standing up or lying down. Ideas are not as easily understood in these positions. Whether we are talking about absorbing, digesting, and assimilating food or ideas, sitting is unique.

If you eat while standing up, your stomach cannot accept the food properly. Standing interferes with the digestive process. When you sit down to eat, you will be more conscious of what you are eating and also how much you are eating. Since sitting is a more relaxed position than standing, you will probably eat less food because you will be digesting what you have eaten more thoroughly and will be satisfied with smaller amounts. When you are seated and you overeat, often you don't know it until you get up from the table. Then you think—oh-oh, I ate too much. In other words, what you are experiencing at that moment of awareness is a natural sensation of fullness. This gives you a gauge by which to measure how much is too much. On the other hand, if you eat standing up, you never know when you've had enough. You lose your natural sense of how much food it takes to satisfy you.

EASTERN AND WESTERN MEDICINE

In the early stages of medicine, during the era of Hippocrates, Eastern and Western medicine were very similar. Both were grounded in practical knowledge and common sense. Both taught the importance of diet and lifestyle in creating good health. In those days, health advice included instructions for properly handling all aspects of life. People were taught to sit up straight when eating and to chew their food thoroughly. These guidelines were considered rudimentary. Then as the East moved toward a more spiritual way of life and the West gravitated toward science and analysis, their commonly held ideas became increasingly divergent. However, certain of these ideas—like sitting down to eat and chewing properly— were passed on from one generation to the next in both the East and the West.

> "Let food be thy medicine, and let medicine be thy food."
>
> —Hippocrates

NOURISHMENT AND BALANCE

Ideally, a meal is a time for nourishing and balancing oneself. A meal is a time to be relaxed, open, and receptive to nourishment, and these attributes don't mix well with activity. Eating while doing other things such as reading, working, watching TV, talking on the phone, or driving interferes with your ability to receive nourishment. Light, quiet conversation is fine because it makes you more open and receptive. (Heavy, loud conversation tightens you up and closes you down.) My analogy is this: If we're talking and in the middle of our conversation I pick up a book, I close off to you. If you're eating, trying to receive nourishment from your food, and you do something else at the same time, you close off to your food. It's that simple. You aren't being fully nourished. Each of us takes different nourishment from the same food. Our ability to receive nourishment depends on how we eat and on our approach to eating.

Many of us don't like to sit down and eat without doing other things, especially when we are alone. When we eat alone, what happens? Thoughts and feelings come up, memories come up. Often we don't like what comes up, but if we learn to think of this as part of a cleansing process, of getting things out that don't belong inside us, it should be easier to eat without distractions. And if we can be patient and allow the unhappy thoughts and feelings to come up, they will be followed by happier ones. In the beginning, just try to let go of your thoughts as you would in meditation. Acknowledge each thought as it comes and then let it pass away.

Food is our strongest desire in life. Food also has the capacity to give us an incredibly deep sense of satisfaction. If we eat quietly and without distraction, we will feel deeply satisfied and fulfilled. However, many people don't allow this to happen. As soon as unhappy feelings come up, they automatically feel the need to do something, to jump up, to read something, to turn on the TV. It's very important to get past this. Let's say that when you begin to practice macrobiotics, you abruptly stop drinking coffee. A headache follows. You can either allow the headache to pass (and the pain might be very intense for a few days) or you can drink a cup of coffee and end it. You might not think so, but this situation is analogous to eating without doing other things. Eating while you distract yourself with something else is the same as taking the very thing (coffee) that was the cause of your problem (headache) in the first place. The cause is also the cure—albeit a very temporary one.

Of all my recommendations, I think sitting down to eat without doing other things is the most difficult one for my clients to practice. At the same time, it's the most important of all the steps. It's the one that sets our direction toward health or toward sickness.

Highlights
- Sitting down to eat your meals and snacks without doing other things is the first step toward good health.
- When you eat without distraction, you absorb the most nutrition.
- You need to concentrate when you read a book or see a movie to get the most out of the experience. You need to participate fully in a conversation to be completely satisfied. This principle applies to your meals as well.
- Sitting down to eat without doing other things allows you to be more aware of what you are eating and to stop when you have had enough.
- You eat less and feel more satisfied.
- This is one of the most difficult steps. Try to always be conscious of it.

Allow adequate time for your meals.
The minimum time required to consume a meal is twenty minutes. Now, you might think that that's an arbitrary number, but it isn't. Let me explain. According to Eastern thinking, everything in the universe is energy, some of it materialized energy (us, for example) and some not (wind, for example). Energy is manifested in vibrations. And we know that vibrations have a natural tendency to align with each other—that's physics. I first realized this when I was in Switzerland, in a shop that sold cuckoo clocks. All the pendulums were exactly aligned. (I was so pleased with my discovery that I made the

mistake of buying one of these clocks. It drove me crazy once I was home.) Or, take the example of women's menstruation. It's well known that after a short while women who share living quarters begin to menstruate at the same time. Therefore, it should not surprise you to learn that after twenty minutes in the same room, the rate of heartbeat, blood pressure, and breathing of those present tends to align. By the same token, if someone should enter the room whose rate of heartbeat, blood pressure, or breathing is very different from that of the group's—too different for alignment to occur—everyone will feel some discomfort, no one will be able to relax completely. Understandably, the person who entered the room will feel too uncomfortable to stay very long.

FIFTY CYCLES OF ENERGY EVERY DAY

Why does the process of alignment take roughly twenty minutes? Here is the reasoning: fifty cycles of energy (*ki*, the Japanese word for energy) flow through the body each day. This means that *ki* circulates through the entire body fifty times a day. One cycle takes just under thirty minutes. It takes seventy percent of the thirty-minute cycle, or about twenty minutes, for alignment to become significant. You can check on this yourself. When you go somewhere new, how long does it take until you really feel comfortable? How long does it take to settle into a serious conversation? It takes about twenty minutes. Still, many people sit down to eat a meal assuming that five to ten minutes is an adequate amount of time. It certainly isn't. If a friend says he has something really important to talk over with you and you say—great, I can give you five minutes—it's likely he or she will feel insulted.

You can't have a serious conversation in five minutes. You can introduce a subject, but you can't delve into it. In the same way, you can have an appetizer or a snack in five minutes but not an entire meal.

Breakfast is the most forgiving meal because we're active for a full day afterward. Dinner is the least forgiving. In other words, if you have a fifteen-minute breakfast, it's not the end of the world. But in a manner of speaking, a fifteen-minute dinner is. It doesn't count as a meal. I'm not talking about solid eating time. I'm talking about the time it takes to complete your meal—from the moment you sit down until the moment you get up from the table.

Let's say you're standing next to someone at a bar. Even if you don't say a word to that person, after twenty minutes your energy will be aligned. If you smile at that person, the alignment happens more quickly. If you talk together, it happens more quickly still and the alignment becomes stronger. I hope you can see now that quiet conversation during mealtimes, talking and eating together, fosters a strong and deep alignment. If you eat quietly without talking, you become more independent, but not as strongly connected to one another. Whether you eat alone or with others, the minimum time for a meal is twenty minutes.

Highlights:
- The minimum time for a meal is 20 minutes.
- Time yourself from the beginning to the end of the meal, not just while you are eating.
- Breakfast is the most forgiving meal in terms of time.

- It takes time for your body to adjust from being active to receiving nourishment, just as it takes time to settle into a good conversation.

Eat slowly and chew well.
It's only common sense that in order to eat slowly you must be seated. You must also allow time in your mind for the meal. If you don't do this you won't be able to slow down. If, when you sit down, you are thinking that you're running late, that you don't have time for this meal, you won't be able to eat slowly. Once you pick up your fork, the pace is set and it's very hard to change it. In other words, eating slowly and chewing well require some preparation.

"Chew your drink, and drink your food."
—Mahatma Gandhi

CHEWING AND POSTURE
In order to chew well, we have to assume the correct posture. The posture for chewing and the posture for reading are exactly the same. If you have something to read that is important to you and requires deep understanding, then you had better sit up straight and tilt your head forward slightly. It is in this position that we can best absorb, comprehend and retain. I think we can agree that if you sit up straight but tilt your chin up slightly, reading becomes more difficult. In order to chew, digest and absorb information completely, we must sit up straight, head tilted slightly forward so the head

spiral is pointing upward. The same holds true if our aim is to circulate, digest and absorb what we eat.

In this position, sitting up straight with your head spiral facing upward, the food remains in your mouth as you chew—it doesn't slip down your throat—and you can circulate (chew) the food as many times as you wish—fifty times, a hundred times, five hundred times. In order to chew thoroughly and well, it's best to put down your utensils between each mouthful and place your hands in your lap. This increases your concentration and encourages thorough chewing.

Why do I place so much emphasis on chewing? Chewing strengthens digestion. If you chew your food well, you will develop your physical ability to digest and assimilate food.

CHEWING AND CIRCULATION

Chewing is a pump. It circulates all our body's energy and fluids, all blood, lymph, digestive, hormonal and cellular fluids. Each chew is like a pump circulating all our energy. Each chew is renewing our physical, emotional, mental and spiritual health. To digest food properly, the minimum count is thirty. To quiet the mind and develop thinking, the minimum is fifty. To refine *ki* (energy), the minimum is one hundred.

In Eastern philosophy, the body is made up of different systems working together and complementing each other. The digestive system and the brain form one of these systems. The digestive system is designed to digest solid and liquid food, the brain to digest vibrational food—food that takes the form of thoughts and images.

CHEWING FOOD—CHEWING IDEAS

Once, while I was living in Japan, I was invited to a restaurant that specialized in *fugu*, a treasured Japanese delicacy. *Fugu* is very expensive. It has a delicious and delicate taste, but it is also highly poisonous. In fact, if it has not been properly prepared, it is usually fatal. Two days before I was scheduled to eat at this restaurant, a famous sumo wrestler died of *fugu* poisoning, a fact which only served to increase my nervousness. But it would have been a terrible loss of face to turn down such an honored invitation, so I went. I drank sake and ate *fugu* with my Japanese friends. None of them seemed unsettled by what had happened to the sumo wrestler, but I wondered if this was to be my last meal. I tried to behave naturally even though I was frightened, and eventually I managed to relax a bit. The *fugu* was delicious. To this day, I don't know whether it was the taste and texture or the danger it posed that made it so interesting to eat.

Later, I told this story to a well-known Japanese macrobiotic teacher, Herman Aihara. He had a good laugh and then said, "A macrobiotic person can't be poisoned. His body won't accept the poison. It will immediately be thrown out of his body. You didn't have to worry."

Maybe, maybe not. But what I do believe is that we can be poisoned by ideas as readily as (or perhaps more readily than) by food. If Eastern thinking is correct about the connection between the brain and the digestive system, then strengthening the digestive system is the easiest way to strengthen thinking ability. In other words, chewing your food and chewing your ideas amount to the same thing. If you chew your food well, you strengthen your ability to digest and assimilate ideas and thoughts. The action of chewing actually improves your thinking ability and your memory. A healthy mind can accept all ideas, chew them over, and either absorb or dispel them. I call this conscious chewing. The concept is applicable to all forms of nourishment, physical, mental, emotional, and spiritual.

CHEWING AND CONSCIOUSNESS

It's important to be conscious of how you eat. Most people eat automatically. They give little or no thought to eating mindfully. Being relaxed before sitting down to eat will help you take the time to chew properly. Doing some stretching, a few yoga postures, or even some deep slow breathing before you start may help you to unwind.

A five-to-ten-minute break between cooking and eating can make a big difference in your ability to enjoy your meal and to concentrate on chewing well. Cooking tends to be tightening and that may contribute to overeating and under-chewing.

You've probably not thought much about chewing. The fact is that most people chew very little. Changing old habits is tough, so before you begin your new program of proper chewing, observe the way you and other people chew. You'll be surprised at what you see and, with a bit of reflection, you'll soon realize that your body deserves better treatment.

Solid food should be chewed until it turns to liquid. Aim to chew each mouthful of food fifty times. Start slowly. For the first two weeks chew each mouthful twenty-five times. Work your way gradually to fifty or, if you have the will and the patience, to a hundred. Once you become accustomed to well-chewed food, you will feel uncomfortable if you eat too quickly.

The more you chew, the more aware you become of your own needs. People today tend to be constantly on the run with little or no time to reflect on what is important to them in their lives. Chewing well will help you break that pattern. It leads naturally to a calmer and more orderly life. By thinking about what's appropriate for you to do next, you will begin to use your time more efficiently; and that, in turn, will help you accomplish more than you ever thought possible.

Everything in Nature occurs in an alternating pattern—movement followed by rest—action followed by inaction. Ideally our lives should reflect this process. We might think we are wasting time if we stop to take care of ourselves and chew our food but, in reality, valuing our quiet time will make our active time more productive.

If you can take at least one or two of your three daily meals alone, you will have the ideal opportunity to concentrate on chewing well. Even if you can chew well at only one meal, you will notice an improvement in how you feel and think. If you can form the habit of chewing well at every meal, your health and your outlook on life will improve dramatically. You can chew well even when dining with others. Take advantage of those times when your companion is talking to do your chewing.

CHEWING AND DIGESTION

Chewing well also releases the full power of saliva. Ideally, saliva has a pH factor of 7.2, which means it is slightly alkaline. Saliva digests complex carbohydrates by breaking them down from complex to simple sugars. (That's why grains, beans, and vegetables get sweeter the longer you chew them.)

Chewing any food well prepares it to pass more smoothly and completely through the digestive system. Saliva can also neutralize imbalances in your food. Even if your diet is not well balanced, thorough chewing helps compensate for the imbalances.

When you chew well, your saliva mixes with the food and makes the food more alkaline, which means the food is better able to absorb the highly acidic secretions that are released in your stomach. If your blood is more alkaline, you will enjoy better health, stronger immunity, and a greater resistance to illness.

Simple carbohydrates and refined foods are absorbed quickly into the bloodstream, creating more acidic blood. Sugar and alcohol are simple carbohydrates. Many foods contain hidden sugar, and sugar can be disguised in various ways on food labels. Most cakes, pastries, cookies, and crackers contain sugar. Fruit is also a simple carbohydrate. Concentrated fruit juices are commonly used as sweeteners in many commercial and health-food-related products. These are all absorbed quickly and they all create acidic blood. Fructose, or fruit sugar, which is found in fruit and honey, can also raise blood cholesterol.

Other foods that are absorbed quickly include white rice, white bread, white pasta, and potatoes. You can help neutralize their acidity by chewing thoroughly, but it's best to avoid these foods altogether once your cravings are minimized.

The problem with these foods is that by the time they reach the stomach, they will have been absorbed in the mucous membranes and therefore will not pass through the duodenum. Foods that are absorbed before passing through the duodenum create more acidic blood. The duodenum has strong alkaline secretions that increase the alkalinity of our food before it passes into the small intestine for final digestion and absorption.

Opposites attract. Chewing alkalizes food. Then the alkaline food attracts stomach acids and the protein content is digested. Food turns alkaline again as it passes through the duodenum where fats are broken down. Your food is then ready for the next stage—final digestion and absorption in the small intestine. Only food that is absorbed through the small intestine creates healthy, alkaline blood. The final stage is water absorption and bowel formation in the colon or large intestine, where the waste products are then excreted.

When your blood is acidic, valuable minerals, especially calcium, are lost from bones, teeth, or muscles. These stored minerals are needed to create the buffer action that breaks down strong acid and turns it into weak acid on its way to being converted to carbon dioxide and water. Mineral loss dilutes the blood and weakens resistance to illness. It weakens the bones as well.

Acid blood weakens the kidneys, heart, and lungs, all organs affected by excessive liquids. The kidneys must work harder to filter more blood and discharge more fluid, which leads to a loss of valuable nutrients (minerals, B vitamins, and vitamin C). The heart has to work harder to pump the increased blood volume. And the lungs must work harder also, in order to discharge the excess carbon dioxide and fluid. Think of the steam that emanates from our mouths when we exhale on a cold day. Think of how much more difficult it is to breathe easily when the weather is humid. Experiment. Try drinking a lot of fruit juice, beer, or soda before exercising. Check your heart and breathing rates and compare the readings with those taken when you drink fewer liquids.

As you can imagine, your health will be adversely affected by a loss of minerals. If you eat a steady diet of refined foods and white sugar, you will weaken your entire system and create a climate for the development of illness.

On the other hand, if you eat foods with healthful, nourishing complex carbohydrates and chew them well, you will enjoy the natural sweetness of good food that can be digested properly. Chewing regulates peristalsis, the automatic expansion and contraction of the muscles of the entire digestive system. Peristaltic movement is wavelike and forms a continuous pattern. Chewing stimulates peristalsis. The more you chew the more frequently the wavelike movement occurs and the more rapidly you move toward a state of balance.

The result is that elimination will return to normal and toxic conditions in the colon, conditions that could cause discomfort and disease, will be warded off. You will have reached the point at which the rhythm of your entire system flows in harmony with the rhythm of Nature and the universe.

Thorough chewing makes the salivary glands produce enzymes that stimulate the release of parotid hormones. These hormones help the thymus gland create T cells, which bolster the immune system.

As I said earlier, chewing also acts as a pump that circulates the body's fluids and energy. Chewing actually activates the blood and other fluid circulation in the body as well as regulating energy flow. If you are feeling physically or emotionally blocked, chewing will help to disperse the stagnation that is causing those conditions. It activates the whole system and dispels negative energy.

BRIGHTEN UP YOUR DAY

After you have chewed thoroughly for a few days or longer, you will notice that you feel brighter and that you are thinking more clearly. This is also easy to test. Try chewing every mouthful of food, even soup and liquids, at least fifty times for four days. Notice the difference. Are you calmer? Is your thinking clearer? Is your energy brighter? If you feel adventurous, try another four days of chewing each mouthful of food at least a hundred times.

To make this a more useful test, it's best to count the number of chews per mouthful over the four-day period. Better chewing alone will strengthen your health but, as I said earlier, make sure that you are seated when you eat and not doing other things—not driving, watching TV, or reading.

RELIEVING STRESS

Most people think they are wasting time when they take time for their meals. The busier and more stressed they are, the more they think they're wasting time. Nothing could be further from the truth. Consider this: the more you rush your meal, the more stressed you become. It's really quite simple. Traditionally there were three times during the day when we stopped what we were doing in order to return to balance, to re-nourish ourselves and readjust our direction. They were called meals—not lunch or dinner breaks—three times a day when we could stop and think, what am I doing, where am I going, what do I want to be doing? If we don't take time for meals, we never develop the ability to ask or answer these questions, and the result is that we lose our direction in life, we lose control over our lives. This is what we see happening today. People are more confused and disoriented than ever before. They never take the time to stop and think about the important things. Meals are purposeful in that they give us the opportunity for this kind of self-reflection. Meals are great stress relievers, provided they are at least twenty minutes long. You will gain time, not lose it, when you take time for your meals.

Highlights:
- Start by chewing each mouthful twenty to thirty times and gradually increase to fifty.
- To improve your health and calm your mind more quickly, chew each mouthful of food at least fifty times.
- Thorough chewing also helps you eat less and feel more satisfied.
- Chewing circulates your body's energy and all its fluids (blood, lymph, hormones, digestive, etc.).
- Put your utensils down after each mouthful. This will help you chew more thoroughly.

Stop eating three hours before bedtime.
"Dine with little, sup with less: Do better still; sleep supperless."
—Benjamin Franklin

Your body cleans and repairs itself while you sleep. Your stomach needs to be empty for this process to be efficient. It takes, on average, about three hours for food to leave the stomach. Therefore, it's best to refrain from eating for three hours before retiring. My analogy is this: It's impossible to clean a room packed with people. If you want to clean a room thoroughly and efficiently, you have to empty it of people. If you want to clean your body, you have to empty it of food.

During the day while we're up and about, we receive the benefits of the sun's energy. Just the opposite occurs at night when we are nourished by celestial energy from the moon, stars, constellations, and galaxy. Daytime is for activity, productivity, and the spending of energy; nighttime is for rest, rejuvenation, and the receiving of energy.

The body cannot perform the miraculous nocturnal task of rejuvenation unless the stomach is empty. Nor can we receive celestial energy at night unless we are empty inside. Food is condensed energy. When you eat, most of your food turns into energy in your body. If you go to sleep too soon after eating, your body will be too full of energy to do its nighttime work. Imagine a roomful of people and then imagine trying to clean, organize, and rearrange that room. Difficult, wouldn't you say? But once the room is empty, it's simple. Can you see from my analogy that your body is in a similar fix if it's not empty? When your stomach is too full, the body is so busy dealing with digestion it can't properly do its normal nighttime job. It's all too easy for the body to fall behind schedule when it can't discharge the toxins that accumulate in our cells and organs each day—which is exactly what happens when it's not allowed to repair itself each night.

HYPOGLYCEMIA

Here's another important point: When we eat, we secrete insulin in order to digest our food. If we eat before sleep, we go to sleep with too much insulin circulating in our bloodstream so that when morning comes, we feel tired and sluggish and have a hard time getting up. This is one of the symptoms of hypoglycemia.

Let me tell you a little bit about hypoglycemia. The food we take before going to sleep is food that the body can't metabolize because it is in a prone position. This food goes to the liver for storage. The liver takes care of fat metabolism, but it also has another important role. The liver neutralizes acidity and therefore helps keep our blood alkaline. When we eat before sleeping, we experience an increased buildup of fat and cholesterol in our bloodstream which, in turn, promotes acidity. And acidic blood is a chief contributor to feelings of fatigue and stress. The excess, undigested food actually exhausts the body, which is unable to process and digest in a reclining position.

Among our vital organs, the liver, pancreas, kidneys, and intestines are particularly overworked. Of course, many people feel they have to eat just in order to sleep. This is a symptom of hypoglycemia. What it means is that your blood sugar has fallen too low for you to fall asleep. Then the body demands that you eat in order to raise your blood sugar level, knowing that it will fall further while you sleep.

Even if what you eat at nine or ten at night is of good quality and healthful, you won't receive the best value from it. It may satisfy your appetite, but without time to digest it properly, you are effectively losing some of its benefits. Foods that are high in fiber and low in fat (e.g., complex carbohydrates) are digested more quickly and easily than animal and dairy foods. They contain less condensed energy and are easier for your body to process and, if you are up and about and active, their energy will disperse more quickly. But even the smallest amount of meat is so laden with condensed energy that it creates an even bigger burden on your body, so much of one that you probably would need more than a three-hour wait before going to sleep.

> "A full belly makes a dull brain."
>
> —Benjamin Franklin

CLEANING YOUR BODY AND BETTER SEX

If you are recovering from an illness, you will benefit from allowing three to four hours of not eating before bedtime. Eating has a nourishing, expansive effect on the body. Cleaning or detoxifying is a process of taking out rather than taking in. Waiting more than three hours before bedtime enhances the body's ability to clean and repair itself during sleep. Experiment with the number of hours you allow yourself between the completion of your meal and your bedtime. When you allow more time, I am sure you will feel the difference the next day. For the record, the suggestion to stop eating three hours before bedtime means you should stop eating three hours before getting into bed or stretching out in a chair with your feet up to watch TV or to read. If your body is horizontal, you haven't complied with the suggestion. You will need to wait an additional three hours if you want to have the best digestion and the best sleep. If you reserve the bed exclusively for sleeping and sex, I'm sure you'll find both activities more rewarding.

> "Eat little, sleep sound."
>
> —Iranian Proverb

Eating before sleep is a hard habit to break. At the same time, you need to realize that you can't have really good health unless you do break it. If you can't go to sleep without eating for three hours beforehand, the most likely cause is that you're not satisfied with the meals you took during the day. The only way to overcome this habit is to make the day's meals more satisfying. Pay particular attention to breakfast, followed by lunch. People who like to be very active and busy don't often sit down for a complete meal during the course of the day. They can't spare the time and they don't want to be slowed down by food. Often they will eat dinner at a very late hour. Whether they eat early or late, this type of person usually feels more relaxed after dinner, and it is this overdue relaxation that stimulates late-night hunger.

Not eating before sleep sounds easy, but it's not. It may require some lifestyle changes.

Highlights:

- To promote the best health, finish your evening meal by eight P.M. Let a full three hours pass before lying down. Stretching out in bed or even on a chaise longue does not allow for good digestion.
- It takes about three hours for your stomach to empty after you finish eating.
- Your stomach must be empty for your body to clean, repair, and recharge itself efficiently while you sleep.
- You will sleep more deeply, need fewer hours, and awake more refreshed.

• Anything you eat before going to sleep—good
food or bad—goes to the liver for storage and
prevents your liver from getting a rest and
repairing itself.

Eat in an orderly manner.
Balance has a certain kind of order. You may think what I am
about to propose is a very rigid way to eat. A number of older
macrobiotic friends have told me just that. My answer is that
I'm still here actively counseling and teaching macrobiotics,
and they aren't. So I'll stick with my way.

What is my way? Let's take dinner: You can start your meal
with soup, followed by a grain and a few different side dishes,
and end it with dessert and/or a beverage, if you choose.

TWO TYPES OF SOUP
There are two main types of soup: savory and sweet. Savory
soups are well seasoned and mildly salty. Their purpose is to
stimulate and activate digestion. Vegetable soup, shoyu soup,
and miso soup (vegetable soup seasoned with miso) are savory.
Among the three, miso soup has the most ability to promote
good digestion.

Sweet vegetable soups are puréed and have a mild, pleasantly
sweet and creamy taste—squash soup, onion, cabbage, and
leek soup, and carrot soup are some examples. The purpose
of sweet vegetable soup is to harmonize, balance, and relax
the digestive system.

Savory soup should be started at the beginning of the meal.
Whether you finish it before going on to the rest of your meal
or continue to consume it throughout the meal, as if it were

a side dish, is up to you. There is actually more benefit in taking this type of soup throughout the meal. Sweet vegetable soup doesn't have the same ability to activate digestion but there's no harm in starting your meal with it. Since it lightens, relaxes, and opens up the digestive system, we can enjoy it throughout the meal as well.

Miso soup is a wonderful way to start the day; however, some people who take miso soup for breakfast can't stop eating all day! It makes them excessively hungry. In those cases, I recommend against it. It's better to take it at lunch or dinnertime. But if you're comfortable with it in the morning and it doesn't cause you to overeat, just keep on with it.

GRAIN FROM BEGINNING TO END

Grain is eaten throughout the meal from beginning to end. Now let's talk about vegetable dishes which are interspersed with the grain. As I said earlier, balance has a certain kind of order. To achieve balance, it's best to follow that order. Take some grain, chew it thoroughly, then move on to the vegetable side dishes. Start with the heavier, long-cooked dishes and finish with the lighter, more quickly cooked ones.

Let's go through the order of a meal together. Start the meal with soup. Then take a mouthful of grain, chew it, and swallow it. If you're having a bean (or bean product such as tofu or tempeh), take that next, followed by another mouthful of grain. Then move on to a sea vegetable, such as hijiki or arame, if you're having one. Take a mouthful, chew that, and swallow it. If you're not quite satisfied by one mouthful of sea vegetable, have another, have two or three if you wish. Take some grain, and then go on to whatever other long-cooked vegetable you may be having. Take another mouthful of grain, and then return to the beans, followed by the long-cooked vegetable, then the grain, and then move on to the more quickly cooked vegetable dishes, those that have been sautéed, steamed, or blanched, for instance. My definition of a lightly or quickly cooked vegetable is this: the crunching sound you make while chewing a lightly cooked vegetable should be audible to the person sitting next to you. No crunch means the vegetable is overcooked. Remember to intersperse the grain with the other dishes. Grain is taken consistently throughout the meal. The salad (pressed salad before raw salad) is taken at the end of the meal. Dessert, if you choose to have one, and tea complete the meal.

A meal eaten in this manner has a wavelike pattern. Think of yourself sitting on the beach, watching the tide go out. The tide doesn't go out all at once, does it? No, it waves out. In other words, it goes out but comes back in a bit, out again but back in a bit, and so on. My point is that although the tide continues to come in, overall it's gradually moving out. In the same way, although grain is taken consistently from the beginning to the end of the meal, overall the meal is moving in a certain direction.

Just to avoid confusion, let me say the following: Adults generally don't finish one dish before going on to the next, but you can if that is your preference. Generally, most children eat through one dish at a time. They like everything to be as simple as possible. Often, they don't like it if the different foods on their plates are even touching. If you wish to develop direct, simple, childlike thinking, you can eat this way. If, however, you want to think more elaborately, then you should move back and forth, in a wavelike pattern. So you are constantly coming back while moving further and further out—like the tide.

Highlights:
- Orderly eating aids digestion and promotes clear thinking. It will leave you feeling more satisfied.
- If you are having soup, start the meal with it. You may finish your soup before going on to the rest of the meal, or you may eat it throughout the meal.
- Eat grains from the beginning to the end of the meal.
- Gradually move from the heavier, well cooked dishes to the lighter, more quickly cooked or raw dishes. Salads come last and are followed by dessert and tea.
- It is not necessary to finish one dish before moving on to the next. The pattern is a wave-like motion that resembles the tide as it goes out.
- Orderly eating leads to orderly thinking.

Avoid mixing foods in the same mouthful.
Keep the foods on your plate distinct and separate, not touching. Imitate the child in this respect. To accomplish this, you either have to take smaller portions or put the different foods in small individual dishes as the Japanese do. I don't like to put everything on my plate at once, so I only take a couple of dishes at a time and then go back for the others. It

often happens that my children finish the foods I like before I'm ready to refill my plate. It's no different when I'm at the Strengthening Health Institute's residential programs. The outcome is that I'm prevented from overeating! Everything is as it should be.

Why do I stress keeping the food on our plates from touching? Digestion is a mechanical process. For instance, if you mix two foods together in the same mouthful, digestive enzymes are going to attach to one food more than to the other. That's their nature. The process works like this: the mouth secretes saliva. Saliva is alkaline. Whichever food becomes more alkalized by the saliva will attract more stomach acid, which, in turn, will attract more alkaline secretions in the duodenum when it arrives there. That food will be well absorbed in the small intestine, and equally so in the large intestine. But the other food will miss out completely. Different foods are digested differently.

If you cook two foods together, such as pressure-cooked rice and beans or stir-fried grain and vegetables, they can be eaten together. They have blended in the cooking process. They are no longer two distinct foods. But if you cook rice and beans separately, eat them separately. Don't put the beans on your rice. There are exceptions. If you cook two dishes separately but mix them together while they're still hot, the residual heat will cause them to blend. In effect, they become one dish. If you want to make a grain and vegetable salad using leftover rice, reheat the rice, then add the vegetables, whether they are raw or previously cooked or freshly cooked. The heat from the rice will allow the ingredients to blend and become digestible. You can let the dish cool down to room temperature before eating it if that is your preference. It is still one dish. Energetically, this is entirely different from mixing distinct foods together on your plate or in your mouth. It's crucial not to mix different foods in the same mouthful. Foods cooked separately should be chewed separately.

As I've already mentioned, children don't like different foods to touch on their plates and, in general, they like simple dishes. But, under some circumstances they do mix everything together. When? When they don't like what they are eating and just want to get it down. When are adults most likely to mix foods together, when they have a healthy appetite and are full of energy, or when their appetite is sluggish and they feel tired?

Here's another question. What stimulates your mind more, eating distinct dishes or eating those that have been mixed together on the plate? The answer, of course, is eating each dish individually. If you eat this way, you will see an improvement in both your digestion and your ability to think.

STEP 2

SET YOUR DAILY SCHEDULE

Rise early and sleep before midnight.
Rise early to be more active and discharge more toxins. The time at which you get out of bed in the morning—not your waking time—is what sets the tone for your day. If you want to be more active and productive, get out of bed by seven A.M. at the latest. If you leave your bed at nine or, even worse, at eleven A.M., there's a sense in which you might as well not bother to leave it at all.

Think about this. The sun rises. It rises with a burst of energy that cleans and refreshes everything on earth. When you get out of bed around the time of sunrise, you can take full advantage of this burst of energy. It is at this time that your body has the greatest capacity to discharge excess, to clean and refresh itself. Within an hour or two after sunrise, the sun's movement starts to slow down. By nine A.M., it has slowed down considerably. Let's take a look at exactly what happens when you get up late, as many people do on Sundays. You have a late breakfast—referred to as brunch—usually sometime between ten and noon, a time when we're meant to be active. Now if we eat when we're meant to be active, we get very sluggish. We lie around for the rest of the day, reading the paper, dragging from one thing to another. The effect on us is the same as if we had overeaten, isn't it? Why should this be the case? The answer is that we don't have the ability to digest or process the sun's energy when we're in a horizontal position. The sun's energy is very coarse. We absorb it through the head spiral located toward the back part of the top of the head, and for this to occur we have to be upright.

If you eat a big meal during the day, afterwards you feel sluggish, you can't think clearly. Even if you take an afternoon nap in a darkened room, you still feel sluggish when you awake. You don't have to be directly exposed to the sun's rays for this to happen. If we are horizontal when the sun is up, we don't have the ability to process the sun's energy. The immune system is effectively deactivated, and the overall effect on us is the same as that of overeating.

It's just as important for our health to be asleep before midnight as it is to rise with the sun. During the night, we receive very subtle energy from the celestial world, the moon, stars, and planets. As we sleep, we are nourished by this celestial influence. We have to be horizontal for this energy to be most effectively absorbed. Our deepest sleep occurs between one A.M. and three A.M. Celestial vibrations are strongest between midnight and four A.M., at the time when the most stars are visible in the sky, the greatest number being visible at about two A.M. It takes an hour or two to fall into the deepest sleep, so we need to be asleep by eleven P.M. to receive the optimal celestial influence and, therefore, the best results for our health. If this is difficult, given the demands of modern society, try to be in bed by midnight.

"Early to bed and early to rise, makes a man healthy, wealthy and wise."

—Benjamin Franklin

I have read that we need a certain number of hours of sleep and if we don't get them, we have to "catch up." If you think about this, it doesn't make much sense. How well or poorly we sleep is determined by our diet and activity during the day. If we eat too much or too little, it's hard to sleep. The same holds true for activity. If we sit around all day, we probably will not sleep well. When we work too hard and exhaust ourselves, sleep often does not come easily. The amount of sleep we need is determined by how long it takes our body to clean, repair, and recharge itself. The better our health, the less time we need for the cycle of cleaning, repairing, and recharging. Most people find that they need considerably less sleep within a couple of weeks of adopting the Strengthening Health recommendations. If our diet and activity are not in balance every day, we won't sleep well at night, and if we don't sleep well at night, our body won't be able to clean, repair, and re-energize its organs and nervous system. On the other hand, if our diet and activity are in balance, the sleeping process becomes very efficient, takes less time to achieve, and gives us deeper sleep. The result is that we feel rested and refreshed with fewer hours of sleep.

If we are in good health, either a rich, elaborate meal or a light, simple one will satisfy us and provide good energy.

The same principle applies to the subject of sleep. The average person in good health requires five to seven hours of sleep. If we get a little less than that, we will still feel fine and, if we choose to sleep a bit longer, perhaps on the weekend, we'll also feel fine. The bottom line is that when we are in good health, we can be flexible about how much we eat and the amount of sleep we need.

Let's consider the quality of sleep. Deep sleep, undisturbed by dreams, is the most refreshing. If you spend the night dreaming, the mind does not have the opportunity to relax and recharge. If you follow the Strengthening Health suggestions accurately, you will not experience confusing or disturbing dreams and you will awaken with the will and the energy to pursue what you want out of life—to pursue your real dreams.

Everyone is concerned with getting a good night's sleep. If you live in proper rhythm with Nature, eat at regular scheduled intervals, chew your food well, and allow enough time before bed for digestion, you will have no problem with sleep.

Highlights:
- Your rising time regulates your energy and activity for the day. Aren't you less productive if you get up late?
- Rise by 7 A.M. to be more active and discharge more toxins. Your body has the greatest ability to discharge and release excess early in the morning.
- Be asleep before midnight to sleep more deeply, awake more refreshed, and be physically stronger.

- Your body can clean and repair itself more efficiently when you are asleep before midnight.

Keep your mealtimes regular.
Regular meals regulate all of your body's cycles—physical, emotional and mental. They make your energy and life more stable. It's important to take your meals at approximately the same time every day. This adjustment alone will greatly improve your health. As easy as this step may sound, the reality is that it takes time and discipline to rethink this aspect of your life. As the world has gotten more complicated, the manner in which we take our most important nourishment is often ignored.

Think about your mealtimes during the past week. Were you able to sit down to your meals at approximately the same time each day? Did you even take the time to sit down when eating breakfast or lunch? If your answer is no, you aren't alone. Most people don't realize the importance of maintaining a regular meal schedule and don't think they are undermining their health by not eating at regular times. But their health is surely suffering.

Even if you still eat meat and potatoes every day, just doing it at regular intervals will let you benefit from your food far more than if you eat these same foods in a disorderly manner. The body responds positively to a set schedule and is very grateful when it is allowed to align itself with Nature—so grateful that it will reward you abundantly with better mental and physical health. This is because the time at which we eat determines how well we digest our food.

When do we have the most active digestion? To answer this question, I have to ask another. Actually, it's a trick question.

Should we eat our meals when we're hungry, or should we eat at regular specified times? The answer is that if we eat regular meals and if we don't overeat, then we will be hungry at mealtimes. Why should this be so?

Aligning with Nature.

Mealtimes are not arbitrary. They are part of the natural cycle of life. Everything in life is governed by the sun's movement, whether throughout the day or throughout the year. The sun has three extreme positions—sunrise, sunset, and the high point in the sky, noon. The extreme angles of the sun indicate what we call mealtimes. The time in between these angles is for activity. Most people are active in the morning and in the spring, less active in the middle of the night or in the dead of winter. Breathing is more active in the daytime and in the summer, and is quieter at night and in the winter.

What breakfast really encourages is rising and separating energy. In the morning, we rise and separate from our families and/or our homes; we all go off in different directions—we separate and enter the larger world. This is the energetic effect of sunrise. We get up, wash, brush our teeth, have breakfast or not, and then leave the house for work, for school, for errands, etc. The usual pattern is one of separating from family and home.

Lunch is a time for either activity or stagnation, depending on when and what we eat. Lunch can give us uplifting, active energy or sinking, stagnating energy. If we want to be active after lunch, we should eat early and the meal should be simple and complete. People who are physically active generally eat a light early lunch. In Spain, lunch is an elaborate meal that is served very late. Since no one can stay awake after such a large and late meal, lunch is quite naturally followed by a long siesta.

Dinner is a time for returning home, a time to gather and unify. Until recently, at least, families ate dinner together, perhaps talking, perhaps arguing, but in any event sharing the events and experiences of the day. Family members communicated, unified, and aligned as a family. This alignment and reunification also follows a natural pattern or tendency.

The nature of energy or of vibrations, as I've mentioned before, is such that vibrations try to align. In other words, they try to become similar in their quality, speed, and direction of movement. Think of a moving merry-go-round. If you want to step on smoothly, you have to be moving in the same direction and at the same speed as the merry-go-round itself. If you are moving faster or slower, your boarding will be jerky because the two different energies are not aligning properly. And, furthermore, should you approach a merry-go-round from the direction opposite to its movement, you will be thrown off even as you attempt to climb on.

Another example of the alignment of energy is this one: Imagine a meeting room filled with vegans who have just finished dinner. Generally, vegans have more peaceful energy because they eat a grain and vegetable-based diet without meat or dairy products. Let's say they drink herbal tea at the end of their meal and as a result are even calmer and more peaceful than usual. In our scenario, these vegans are discussing various types of meditation when someone new enters the room, momentarily disrupting the conversation. Let's say that the newcomer has just left the local sports bar, where he has eaten a dinner of fried chicken washed down with a few beers. The atmosphere in the bar was heated because the local hockey team was losing. You can appreciate that this person's energy would be very strong, perhaps even jarring, compared with the energy of the vegans. The group would no doubt lose its focus and wonder who this guy was and why he was there. Do you see the problem? The newcomer's energy is just too different for it to align quickly with the energy of the others. Either the newcomer or the vegans will feel uncomfortable. Only as time passes will their energy even start to align.

When members of a family come together on a daily basis, they build understanding and communication. So long as they do this, the family will function harmoniously. Each of us goes out every day and encounters many different influences and experiences. We eat different foods, talk to different people, engage in different activities, all of which alter our condition and thinking. We align with individuals outside the family through common or similar points and qualities. This is not a threat to the family, but an asset—as long as we continue to take our evening meal together. Understanding and communication develop as we talk and eat together. We can go out again after dinner, if we choose. As long as the unification process, the aligning process continues at the evening meal, the family's stability and balance will develop and be maintained.

Breakfast, Lunch, and Dinner.

Now that we know that meals are meant to align us with Nature's energy, let's talk specifically about breakfast, lunch, and dinner. As I said earlier, breakfast should give us rising and separating energy so that we can be in harmony with the natural world. The sun rises, the dew evaporates, flowers open. Breakfast the world over has one ingredient in common, and that is liquid. When, for instance, we boil water for tea or coffee, the boiling water evaporates, creating rising and separating energy. Whether breakfast consists of cold cereal with milk, porridge (the difference between a macrobiotic person's breakfast grain and dinner grain is simply the amount of liquid used), miso soup, orange juice, coffee, tea, or simply a glass of water, liquid is the common ingredient. It is what we need to rise and separate. A breakfast consisting of bacon, eggs, and dry toast makes for a difficult day. The food is too dry to create active, separating energy. If we want to get moving, we would have to spread some jam on our toast and have a glass of juice or a cup of coffee. It's the liquid that enables us to be active in the morning. If breakfast is too dry, we're not able to align with Nature's rising and separating energy. On the other hand, we can still function perfectly well if we take just liquid for breakfast.

Breakfast time is also the time to separate from home. If you work at home and don't leave the house before you settle down, if you go from your bed to your office or your studio, perhaps by way of the bathroom and kitchen, I think you'll find that after a while you lose your creativity and your drive. There is simply no polarity. If you work at home, my suggestion is that you go out and do something, then return. Have a cup of tea, buy a newspaper, or just take a walk around the block. Unless you have some degree of separation after breakfast, you'll find that you become tired and stale as the morning wears on.

Dinner is a different matter. Dinner should be more substantial—longer-cooked and not too watery—too much liquid can interfere with sleep. If at dinner we drink too much beer, wine, apple juice, soda, coffee, or tea—the common point being liquid—we can't sleep. (Sugar changes to water in the body, which means we have to watch our intake of simple carbohydrates also.) Dinner should give us settling down and gathering energy since it coincides with the setting of the sun. Dinner is the most suitable meal at which to have a protein.

Imagine your day if you swapped breakfast and dinner. You could no longer align with Nature's energy. Mealtimes are not arbitrary, as I said earlier. The meal is our way of aligning with Nature's energy no matter where we are—even if we live in the middle of Manhattan in a high-rise made of materials that carry an incredible electromagnetic charge, a place where we couldn't be more isolated from Nature. If we have regular meals that consist of appropriate ingredients for the time of day, we will be able to align with Nature's energy. By contrast, if we live in the most pristine setting and eat chaotically, we may be surrounded by Nature but we are not aligning with it. Meals create our connection to Nature. I think of the meal as an anchor that creates stability in our lives, no different from the anchor that keeps a ship from drifting into dangerous waters.

Lunch. Around lunchtime, the sun climbs to its highest point in the sky and appears to hang there motionless for a while before it begins its descent. There are two sorts of energy to choose from at lunchtime: one is active energy, the other is more stagnant. If you want to be active and productive in the afternoon, you would be wise to eat while the sun is still rising. If you wait to eat until it's hanging out at its high point, your energy for the afternoon will be more stagnant.

If we want to be active in the afternoon, at what time should we begin lunch? To answer this question, let's go back to the example I gave earlier. Think about the after-lunch siesta for which Spain is famous. When is lunch eaten in Spain? Usually, from two to four P.M. At twelve, should they even be open, the restaurants are empty. Portugal and Spain are next door to one another, but Portugal has no siesta. In Portugal, lunch is eaten either from twelve to one P.M., or from one to two P.M. During the tourist season, you can distinguish the Spanish from the Portuguese simply by the times they choose to eat. The Portuguese are leaving the restaurants as the Spaniards are entering. The different dining habits of these two cultures are emblematic of their different lifestyles. Nevertheless, in spite of the late hours at which they dine, Spaniards still rise with the sun and therefore enjoy long and productive mornings.

So, if you want to be active in the afternoon, finish lunch by two P.M. at the latest—one P.M. would be even better. The later you start lunch, the less you can accomplish afterwards. It's as simple as that. Remember that when you eat, you are aligning with the sun's energy. Try this test. Eat similar lunch food every day for four weeks, but for the first two weeks start lunch at twelve P.M. For the following two weeks, start it at two P.M. You will certainly notice a difference. It's common knowledge that the best way to ensure being useless in the afternoon is to eat a late, rich lunch.

Lunch should be simple yet complete and satisfying. Think of foods that allow you to remain physically and mentally active. The test is whether or not you can work, think, and be productive after eating them. Here are a few possibilities using grains or grain products and quickly cooked vegetables: vegetable sushi rolls (brown rice and vegetables wrapped in toasted nori seaweed), rice balls, fried rice, fried noodles or noodles in broth, and quick-steamed vegetables or vegetable sautées. What qualifies as a simple and complete meal in our part of the world? The sandwich does. Sandwiches are simple and quick and can be complete and healthful, depending on what's in them. Tofu, hummus, or any vegetable-type spread served on steamed and un-yeasted sourdough bread is an example of a nourishing sandwich. You can complement the sandwich with a bowl of vegetable soup and a vegetable side dish, a salad, for instance. Not so long ago, a lunch consisting of a bowl of soup, a sandwich, and a pickle was a fairly typical meal.

MEALTIMES

Should the main meal of the day be served at midday, or at sunset? Well, there's a good argument for both. Agrarian societies took their main meal at noon and ate lightly in the evening. The advent of the Industrial Age changed that, because a simple meal fit in better with the workday. Both will produce good health; choose what suits your lifestyle.

Try not to skip any meals. How much you eat is up to you; what is significant is the regularity. If you cannot make every meal regular, the most important one is your main meal of the day. Having a regular dinner, the gathering, unifying meal, provides the most benefit. When I say a meal should be served at the same time every day, I mean it. A fifteen-minute variation in the schedule is acceptable. Thirty minutes is pushing it. Remember that mealtimes regulate all your body's cycles, so the timing is important for your health.

Your blood-sugar level is one function that follows the sun's movement, as do your activity and energy levels. Digestion, bowel movements, all of your physical and mental cycles— they, too, follow the sun's movement. So if you want regular digestion, regular bowel movements, regular menstruation, regular blood-sugar levels, and more balanced emotions, sit down to regular meals.

When I lived in Portugal, I spent a lot of time in the company of old friends who had been living there for a number of years. We shared many meals together. In some ways, they were more careful about what they ate than I was. Yet that family—both parents and children—did not enjoy good health. I believe there was a single reason. Even though they ate good-quality food, they never sat down to regular meals. They ate when they were hungry, and often they ate standing up.

Nothing has a stronger effect on regulating the body's cycles than regular meals. And nothing has a more disruptive effect than skipping meals, eating chaotically, or eating erratically.

The starting times for our three regular meals are as follows: Breakfast, five A.M. to eight-thirty or even nine A.M. Lunch, eleven A.M. to one P.M. Dinner, five P.M. to seven or even seven-thirty P.M. The time at which we eat determines how well or poorly we digest our food. The above are the times at which we have the most active digestion, the times at which we can digest our food most thoroughly. The principle behind this applies to sleep as well. Let's say you need six hours sleep a night. Which schedule will give you more energy: sleeping from eleven P.M. to five A.M., or sleeping from three to nine A.M.? Clearly you are much better off sleeping from eleven P.M. to five A.M., rising when the sun rises to take full advantage of the sun's energy.

Highlights.

- Regular meals regulate all your body's cycles, physical, emotional, and mental.
- You will have better energy and digestion, more regular moods, and clearer thinking.
- The time you start your meal regulates your metabolism. Start your meals earlier to be more active and productive. Breakfast: five to eight-thirty A.M. (nine A.M. at the latest). Lunch: eleven A.M. to one P.M. Dinner: five to seven P.M. (seven-thirty P.M. at the latest).
- Your health will improve more quickly and be more stable.
- Eat your meals at the same time every day.

THE BRIEF HISTORY OF FOOD

Food nourishes us and is necessary to sustain life, but it is also much more than that. A meal is actually about taking the time to receive life. It is the counterbalance to work, exercise, and creative expression. When we take our meals, we realign with Nature and with each other. Most importantly, meals are a time for receiving rather than giving. We exchange ideas and share socially. This is how we return to balance.

How we look at and relate to food itself has changed dramatically over the last 12,000 years of recorded history. The changes have come largely due to the development of an agrarian civilization that eventually gave way to one dominated by science, technology, and industry. It has only been in recent centuries in the West, and now globally, that human beings have begun to feel entirely separate from each other and from Nature.

Macrobiotics, as we know it today, developed during the 20th century in an effort to integrate the spirituality that developed in the East with the modern science and technology that was developing in the West. George Ohsawa, the founder of modern day macrobiotics, synthesized these ideas from traditional understanding and coined the word macrobiotics to mean "life according to the largest view." Michio and Aveline Kushi, along with others of George Ohsawa's students, further developed and refined these ideas and then applied them to improving the health and way of life in modern society. Michio Kushi defined macrobiotics as "the universal way of health and longevity."

Macrobiotics is neither a traditional way of eating, nor is it a Japanese diet. It is traditionally based; the modern macrobiotic diet and lifestyle practices developed out of and evolved from the diet and lifestyle practices of the peoples and cultures of the world's long-standing civilizations. The macrobiotic diet incorporates the world's most unique foods from these civilizations (such as rice and miso from Asia, and sourdough from Europe, sesame tahini from the Middle East, peanut butter from the West, etc.) and uses them often or daily. Macrobiotic principles are expressed in the traditional cuisines of Asia, India, the Middle East, Europe, and Africa. My understanding and research has shown me that all the world's long-standing civilizations were grain and vegetable-based, all of them had a very strong sense of place, culture, identity, and connection to Nature, and therefore were all, in fact, macrobiotic.

As the 21st century unfolds, we continue to increase our involvement in food production and systems. The lifestyle practices of macrobiotics are useful and spiritually fulfilling. They help us learn how to realign with Nature and with those parts of ourselves we feel we may have lost in the past century.

THE BRIEF HISTORY

~12,000 years ago—retreat of the last Ice Age in northern Europe.
Previously, food was scarce and modern agriculture was yet to
be rediscovered. Around this time, two noteworthy developments occurred: significant developments in agriculture and
strides in boat building occurred over the next few thousand
years, which paved the way and made possible our modern
society. People could now stay in one place and more easily
interact with neighboring people.

~10,000 years ago—evidence of agricultural villages.
The cultivation of cereal grains and the advent of modern
grains such as barley, millet, wheat, and rice coincided with
the domestication of animals as well as the development of
pottery and weaving. The agricultural revolution led to the
development of villages.

All the world's long-standing civilizations cultivated grains
as the principal food upon which every meal was based. Over
time, people have become synonymous with and inseparable
from their grains: rice in the Orient, bulgur, couscous, pita
in the Middle East; chapatti in India; bread in Europe; oats
in Britain; corn in the Americas. For example, you cannot
separate rice from Asia, bread from Europe, or corn from the
Americas.

There is a format to a meal. Whereas the food pyramid
makes recommendations based on a total daily intake of
certain foods, it is much more helpful to plan eating around
individual meals. A basic macrobiotic meal includes a grain,
and at least one separate vegetable dish. A bowl of soup may be

taken at one meal each day. Meals made primarily of grains, beans, vegetables, soup, and pickled and fermented foods remained largely unchanged for thousands of years. Chiefly supplemental to grains, beans, vegetables, and soups were animal and dairy foods. Historically, in agricultural societies, these foods were eaten in surprisingly small quantities. Meat and dairy were supplemental, not principal foods. Meat was eaten primarily at special feasts and celebrations. In more extreme climates and mountainous regions, dairy products were often used in ways similar to the use of miso and shoyu (fermented soybean products) in Asia.

~ *2,000–3,000 years ago—ancient Greece and Rome began introducing the foods, cuisines, sweets, and spices from their trades with and conquests of tropical and sub-tropical areas.*

~*500–600 years ago—age of exploration, trade, and expansion rapidly increased the availability and popularity of exotic foreign foods and vegetables, sugar and spices, plants, and cooking styles.*

During the beginning of the age of western exploration and expansion in the 15th and 16th centuries, foods that were once locally grown and indigenous to other parts of the world became more widely distributed. Tropical fruits and vegetables became more widely cultivated with their rise in popularity for customary table fare. For instance, the Spanish brought the potato (indigenous to Chile and the Andes) to Europe. Once in Europe, the potato gained wide acceptance over the next two hundred years. This starchy nightshade (related to tomatoes, peppers, and eggplants) began to replace the cereal grains in other cultures. Together with the tomato, these two foods "conquered" Europe more thoroughly than any other. With the age of exploration and western expansion, many diets lost the important indigenous connection to food, which confused alignment with and created separation from Nature's cycles.

~300–200 years ago—The Industrial Revolution.
Britain, Europe, and the United States began adapting from an agrarian to an industrial society.

~90–100 years ago—World War I
Advances made in nutritional studies and food science.

~80–70 years ago—World War II
Food science proliferated. The USDA Basic 7 Food Groups recommended that animal and dairy foods comprise about one quarter of the American Diet to keep us strong and healthy. Chemicals were introduced into agriculture and the food supply. Modern food preservation also proliferated.

The Industrial Revolution in the 18th and 19th centuries had the greatest effect on changing the eating patterns that led to the modern diet. The industrialization of Britain, Europe, and the United States ushered in technological advances that enhanced the general quality of life as well as agricultural productivity. Industrialization created a demand for people to migrate to cities as well as implementing the widespread construction of factories. Transportation and communication were more mobile, but migration from rural to urban life affected people's eating habits—including dietary proportions.

Daily life became further removed from the natural cycles of the sun, moon, and seasons, and instead began to conform to a business week and a weekend. Nutrition became more imbalanced. With the new pressures of modern, industrialized life, slowly, physical and mental degenerative diseases began to increase.

Refined foods, especially refined grains, became more available on a wider scale (flour, for example, now could be sifted, easily packaged and ready-to-use, whereas, previously, time was needed to prepare the flour at home by hand). Refined foods, however, cause a nutritional imbalance, and many refined foods also cause blood to become more acidic. Minerals create a buffer action to neutralize the acidity. Refined grains lack these minerals. The greatest stores of minerals in grains are in the bran, which is partially or completely removed in the refinement process. Nutrition itself is a fine balance, where one nutrient is needed to absorb and utilize another. Altering this natural balance easily creates an excess of certain nutrients and a deficiency of others.

The combination of the disruption of eating patterns and the addition of refined grains caused nutritional imbalances and deficiencies. Refined grains allowed for the increased use of animal and dairy foods. We crave to supplement the nutrition lost in the refinement process. Increased animal and dairy foods in turn increase our cravings for sweets. These changes largely contributed to the vicious cycle that is the trademark of the modern diet—a diet high in refined foods, animal and dairy fats, and sweets. The strain of modern degenerative diseases began around the beginning of the 20th century and increased following World War II.

In the early 20th century, food began to be broken down into its components: calories, vitamins, proteins, minerals, etc. Judging food based on its components not only perpetuated imbalance, it helped create it. To break down food into its components is to take Nature out of food. Between WWI and WWII, recommendations to increase the consumption of animal and dairy protein only added to the confusion.

WWII paved the way for more devastating changes to our food supply as well as to our nutritional guidelines. Modern, commercial food preservation is a by-product of WWII when methods were developed to ensure that foods would last for an indefinite period of time for soldiers overseas. This form of preservation prevents oxidation, enzymes, or bacteria from changing the food in any way. Chemical preservatives take life out of the food, making "dead foods" that cannot sustain health.

The uniqueness of food is that it is always different. The same dish cannot be made twice. Living foods change. Traditional methods of preservation such as drying, smoking, pickling, fermenting, and cold storing maintain and improve the nutrition available in the food, while simultaneously enhancing the natural quality. For example, sun drying increases vitamin D in mushrooms the same way it does in our own skin. Natural pickling and fermentation produces digestive-aiding enzymes, unique and previously nonexistent nutrients, and vitamin B-12. Storage apples increase in both taste and nutrition. Un-yeasted sourdough bread is another example of a traditional preparation that enhances nutrition and satisfaction. Eating naturally preserved foods also enhances our own ability to synthesize nutrients we need. These foods are still living and slowly undergo subtle changes.

Frozen fruits and vegetables also increased during the period after the war. Analytically, these foods may be similar to fresh produce, but our bodies cannot be fooled. Nutrition is more than what can be measured in a laboratory.

Lastly, but not least, chemicals found their way into agricultural production. The chemical industry developed to create munitions for the war effort. Prior to WWII, natural foods were still commercially available. Whole-grain breads, untreated, local vegetables, natural pickles, and animals raised without hormones and antibiotics were still largely available. However, following the war, the chemical products were immediately applied to agriculture. Petroleum-based fertilizers began their widespread use after WWII. Slowly, the soil changed from living matter, teeming with and supportive of life, to inert matter.

"A nation that destroys its soils destroys itself.
Forests are the lungs of our land, purifying the
air and giving fresh strength to our people."
—Franklin D. Roosevelt

The excessive use of these fertilizers has destroyed living matter across countless acres of soil and has transformed this soil into inert matter made up of petroleum and its byproducts. This destruction causes further soil erosion and ultimately these chemicals seep into our water supplies. The soil on commercial farms is more closely related to plastic, chemically speaking, than soil. This type of soil can only produce lifeless foods. The loss of minerals, unique microorganisms, and other life produces weak crops that need the aid of weed and pest killers in order to live long enough to harvest. These additional chemicals further weaken the crops, and our immune systems along with them.

Note that crop losses have increased each passing year since the late 1940s. This loss is proportional to the increased use of chemicals in agriculture. The soil is not very different from our collective immune systems. Our immunity has further decreased with the excessive use of antibiotics.

We have truly entered the era of modern degenerative illness. We are now expected to die of a degenerative illness, especially heart disease, cancer, or diabetes if an accident does not claim us first. Modern giant food companies have made a science out of food so that it is now possible to create it in a laboratory. It was in the era of WWII that our perception of food as something whole and unique was altered, broken up and transformed into a series of nutrients that could be measured and given out. As a result, food in the modern age is one hundred percent consistent, but that also leads to the conclusion that it is not food at all.

~1953 TV became more popular and Swanson introduced TV Dinners.

~1955 First McDonald's opened.

~1956 The USDA modified nutritional recommendations to The Basic Four.

The Basic Four recommended animal and dairy foods to comprise as much as 50% of diet, which changed the way the entire world eats.

The diet and food quality in the West further deteriorated after fast foods appeared in the 1950s. Complete meals could simply be heated at home in the oven for a few minutes. The original fast-food restaurants began their spread throughout the United States and Britain. By the 1970s, fast foods had taken over completely. This coincided with the break from the traditional values of the society. Seemingly hundreds and thousands of years of tradition disintegrated overnight.

Most people born since the end of WWII no longer remember what fruits and vegetables are; they have been largely forgotten. Grains were grouped together with potatoes and reduced to starches. The trademark of the modern diet became meat and potatoes. The mythology that complete chains of amino acids could only be found in animal and dairy foods persisted until the 1970s. Although Frances Moore Lappe in her book *Diet for a Small Planet* dispelled this mythology, she still allowed the idea that protein-based nutrition was important.

All food has protein. We do not need to emphasize protein in our diet. The combination of grain, beans, vegetables, seeds, nuts, and fruits gives us the ideal amount of protein to promote lasting health. But the most important thing is that the body runs on glucose, which comes from the complex carbohydrates in our diet. The most important complex carbohydrates are unrefined grains, beans, and land and sea vegetables. What you eat today becomes your blood plasma tomorrow. Our blood plasma renews itself every ten days. We don't need to think of our food combining for complete proteins as long as we eat a variety of these complex carbohydrates within ten days.

> "If man's Soul is indeed a kind of Stomach, what else is the true meaning of Spiritual Union but an Eating together?"
>
> —Thomas Carlyle

Sadly, the family meal began to disappear with the new ease of getting quicker and seemingly more efficient meals. It fit in perfectly with the modern technological lifestyle. The family meal is the "glue" of a society. It provides a sense of belonging and stability in life. The dinner meal is very important because it gives everyone a chance to reunite and share the experience of food. Now that the family meal has dissolved, order has begun to change. Recent research has shown that one meal a day that includes talking with each other increases a child's chance of going to college as well as their ability to avoid drugs and alcohol. Cooking with electricity saved time, and getting a meal on the table became even more convenient when the microwave oven was introduced. Both have lessened our sensitivity to food and to cooking.

This is the completion of a cycle. Food that was once natural and shared for proper physical, emotional, and spiritual nourishment and social enjoyment has deteriorated to an almost careless, mechanical process or afterthought.

The modern meal as we know it does not fit into a busy schedule. The demands of today's business world are so intense and so overwhelming that we cannot take the time to stop work and eat properly. We have lost touch with Nature and our ability to respond to the changing seasons. We are losing touch with our true human nature, and our feelings are confused. We can no longer enjoy and be guided by the natural rhythms of life.

~2008 *The recession and banking collapse.*
People are becoming more self-reliant, which includes taking responsibility for our own health.

~2009 to the present day—the continuing development of local food communities.

The 21st century presents us with many choices and opportunities to either continue along a path toward illness or move in the direction of health, both for ourselves and the planet. We are in a unique era when history and science have the opportunity to support each other to create a new medicine for humanity. We can start to move toward health when we reestablish connections to each other, to our communities, to Nature, and to the planet. Now more than ever, science confirms and validates parts of the human experience that have passed the test of time. A healthy future depends on both personal and planetary health.

The recession in 2008 was different from others. For all of my time involved with health, a recession characteristically causes people to spend more time and money on their health. Since 2008, people have been diverted from investing in their personal health. Due to environmental and societal pressures, getting through the day seems to be the main priority of many people. At the same time, there is a counterbalance to this.

"Though an old man I am but a young gardener."
—Thomas Jefferson

We are experiencing a broader collective desire for, and a return to, a local slow-foods culture. Vegetables are in vogue. Farmers' markets and CSAs are gaining momentum and spreading throughout the country. "Go Green" is a marketing and branding mantra. Artisanal and fermented foods are now becoming a lucrative entrepreneurial niche in some communities. Preserving biodiversity through collecting seeds on small farms and exchanging them with others is now once again an operating prerogative of the true organic agriculture in the country.

In some ways, we seem to have returned to some of the natural philosophies held by the founding fathers. Ben Franklin and our early presidents placed great value in preserving land, seed, and agricultural systems. They were aware of the importance of our connection with Nature and the land. They shared a vision of building a nation and wealth based on an agrarian society, that personal and environmental health were interrelated.

Two understandings are now more widely accepted than they have been for decades. The first understanding is that there is a direct relationship between diet and health. The second is that there is a direct relationship between our food choices and the environment, including climate change. Our awareness and respect for all aspects of life is beginning to grow again: for Nature, for the climate, for animal rights, for our collective future on this planet.

I see the practice of macrobiotics as a creative hub for the 21st century. A diet and lifestyle that helps to integrate our spiritual perceptions about the world around us, as well as the practical integration of a sustainable agriculture that promotes healthy people and a healthy planet. We all have a vital role in creating personal and planetary health through our daily choices. Step 3 demonstrates some practical applications to make this possible.

DIET:
CONTENT AND QUALITY
OF MEALS

EAT TWO OR THREE COMPLETE AND NUTRITIONALLY BALANCED MEALS EVERY DAY

Grain and vegetable dishes together at the same meal provide the most complete and balanced nutrition.

> "A meal without a grain is just a snack."
> —Michio Kushi

PLAN EVERY MEAL AROUND COOKED GRAINS AND GRAIN PRODUCTS.

Moses in the desert

Let's look at the biblical story of Exodus. Moses took the Jewish people out of Egypt to deliver them from slavery into freedom. He wanted the Jews to build a new life free of the old enslaving concepts. However, the elders preferred what they knew to the possible dangers of the unknown. To fulfill his dream, Moses elected to have his people wander in the desert for forty years until the older generation died off. By then, the young had grasped the idea of living in freedom.

We have reached the end of a long dietary journey into the desert which emphasized animal and dairy foods as the basis of healthy meals.

The largest error was to assume that science was superior to Nature, as you found at the beginning of this section in the Brief History of Food. One significant myth was the notion that cow's milk or infant formula was healthier for babies than mother's milk. I was part of that experiment. My mother didn't nurse me. She fed me commercial baby formula followed by cow's milk. When I was in my twenties and learned about the physiological and psychological benefits of nursing for both mother and child, I asked her why she hadn't nursed me. She answered simply that at the time, doctors thought bottle-feeding was superior. Now we know that nursing develops children's immunity, general health, and thinking ability. It also helps children feel more secure emotionally and promotes a deeper bond between mother and child than bottle-feeding.

Maybe your parents and grandparents started the day with a bowl of oatmeal, barley, Wheatena, Cream of Wheat, or corn grits. Compare that practice with today's choice of bacon and eggs with white toast, bagels with cream cheese, or coffee with doughnuts and/or muffins. Many people ate beans and a variety of seasonal fresh vegetables. Vegetable soup was considered essential daily fare. Yes, people did consume some animal and dairy food, but usually in small portions and balanced by all the fresh, natural food in their diets. Even common snacks that people once enjoyed, such as seeds, nuts, and dried fruits have been more or less forgotten. And, in many parts of the country, anyone advocating healthful food choices is thought to be referring to some foreign diet.

Macrobiotics is a way to help integrate these foods we forgot in the desert.

Today, the current recommendations strongly resemble the Healthful Foods List in the back of this book. This proves that there is a new awareness about healthful nutrition. Hopefully, the government will realize soon enough that plant protein is superior to animal protein and we have no need for dairy food after we are weaned from our mother.

> "Healthy citizens are the greatest asset any country can have."
>
> —Winston Churchill

Cereal Grain

There is one major problem, however. Hardly anyone today knows what a cereal grain is (cereal grain was the traditional name for all grains). If you ask people whether they eat cereal grains, the likely answer will be yes. That's because most of us think that dry breakfast cereals such as Cheerios, Rice Krispies, and corn flakes are cereal grains. To avoid confusion, I use the word "grain" to mean cereal grains that have been boiled, pressure-cooked, or used in traditional breads.

So let's talk about grains. Basically a grain is made up of three parts:

- Bran, the outer layer of the kernel, is the part that protects the grain from oxidation. It contains protein, minerals, and vitamins.

- Germ, the heart of the life-giving part, contains oil and vitamins. It is actually the seed of the grain.
- Endosperm, the starchy bulk or center of the grain, is mostly carbohydrate. It is the fruit of the grain, the food the seed uses to grow.

A single grain contains the beginning and the end of all plant food, since it merges the seed and the fruit into one. Grains and grain products are either "whole" or "refined." A grain is whole when all three of those parts are undisturbed and complete. A grain is refined when part or all of the bran or germ has been removed. The more of the bran and germ that is removed, the more refined the grain is. The more refined the grain, the more out of balance it is and the less nutritional value it has. Rice, wheat, and corn are the principal grains grown for human consumption. Rice is used by more than half of the world's population and is seen most widely in one of two types—brown rice and white rice.

Brown rice is whole-grain rice, with only the husk removed; it can be bought in any of three forms—short, medium, or long grain. Short and medium-grain rice are more natural to temperate climates; long-grain rice is preferable in hotter climates. Short-grain rice has more of a glutinous quality (not to be confused with the gluten in wheat), and when cooked it is somewhat stickier than long-grain rice. Brown rice is the world's most balanced food and is extremely high in nutritional value. It is recommended to be eaten often or daily. Brown rice combines deliciously with all other foods, even foods that are not part of the macrobiotic diet. Amazingly, whatever is cooked in the same pot with brown rice will be thoroughly cooked in the same amount of time it takes to cook the rice.

White rice has had its bran and germ removed, so it does not begin to compare nutritionally with brown rice. You would have to eat seven times as much white rice as brown to ingest the same nutrients!

Referring to a familiar, everyday food such as rice as a "grain" seems to confuse people. Virtually everyone has eaten lots of rice over the years, but probably without ever thinking of it as a grain. Rice is readily available and simple to cook, and it's important that you make it a staple of your daily diet.

Another excellent way to ensure that your meal revolves around a grain is to eat pasta or noodles as your main food. Most people tend to like pasta. I am referring, of course, to good quality pasta or noodles, such as Italian durum wheat semolina pasta or Japanese udon or soba. Later in the book you will find a list of other grains, some of which are probably unfamiliar to you. It's best to start by eating brown rice and to develop the habit of making grains the focus of your meal.

When you are ready, visit the natural-food section of your local supermarket or health-food store and check out the grains. Incorporate those you are already familiar with into your diet. If they are already part of your diet, use them more regularly as the centerpiece of your meals. My suggestion is that you plan every meal around cooked grains and grain products. Then complete and balance every meal with one or two vegetable dishes. Activate and harmonize your digestion with a bowl of vegetable soup at one or two meals. And always buy the highest-quality organically grown, unrefined, and naturally processed foods you can find.

Grains and vegetables at every meal

Just as we use our mealtimes and rising and sleeping times to align externally with Nature's cycles, so we use the meal itself to align internally with our own biological cycles. Ongoing alignment with both cycles creates a powerful environment for the development of spiritual, emotional, and physical health. We cannot create this important biological alignment without first defining what we mean by the word "meal." A meal consists of a grain or grain product and at least one separate vegetable dish. Even if the grain or grain product has many vegetables in it, such as stir-fried noodles and vegetables, it is classified as a grain dish. This being the case, we are still missing a separate vegetable dish. When we add the vegetable dish, we have a meal. What I'm saying is this: your vegetable dish needs to be a separate dish, not vegetables cooked in or with something else, for example, in soup or in grains or grain products. Any vegetable cooked with grain becomes part of the grain dish. Any vegetable cooked in soup becomes part of the soup itself. To be annoyingly clear about this: the essence of a meal is a grain or grain product and at least one separate, standalone vegetable dish.

> "Tell me what you eat, and I will tell you what you are."
>
> —Anthelme Brillat-Savarin

Principal foods

The term "principal food" refers to the food that is the centerpiece or core of the meal. In the modern American diet, protein in the form of meat or poultry or fish has been the most common principal food. In today's world, when a meal is planned, the first decision to make is what protein to serve. The rest of the meal evolves from this starting point. Most of the world's longstanding cultures, however, planned their meals around the grain dish, and this is the format we use. The first question to ask is: "What grain or grain product will be the centerpiece of my meal?" We might choose brown rice, barley, noodles, good-quality bread, polenta, or cracked wheat. The choice of grain is the center point around which the rest of the meal—which should include vegetables and other supplemental foods—should be planned.

The point is that natural foods, such as grains and vegetables, which all bestow health benefits, have been out of the mainstream American diet for such a long time that they are now considered weird. If you mention the word rutabaga or parsnip, most people don't know if you're talking about a vegetable or a dance craze. I recently heard of a family in which the children actually used the word rutabaga to taunt and insult each other! We have gotten so far away from wholesome food that we as a nation need reeducation. Paradoxically, although we live in a high-tech world that requires us to master very complicated material, for many of us the thought of having to acquire the simplest, most basic knowledge—how to improve our health through healthful eating—is overwhelming.

Cooking classes are the best starting place for your reeducation. Check the bulletin board of your natural food store for information on cooking classes, lectures or seminars on natural diet and lifestyle. While you are there, pick up a cookbook or two. Cookbooks are good for ideas and inspiration once you have an understanding and image of healthful cooking and eating.

In the beginning stages, cooking can be learned only through personal experience. This is true of any style of cooking. To learn how to make a dish, we need to know three things—how the dish should look, how it should taste, and how it should smell. We cook from an image, and these factors form the basis of the image of whatever we are making. Once we have an image, we can reproduce the dish. If, when eating out, I come across a dish that I particularly like, I often replicate this dish at home—with slightly different ingredients, if necessary—but the point is that I always work from an image to create a new and healthful addition to my family's diet. In the past, people cooked using their intuition rather than cookbooks; but many years of eating foods that do not properly nourish the brain or the spirit have hampered our intuition.

A Great Way to Eat Food

"Macrobiotics is a great way to eat food." This is the answer given by my son Joe to the question, "What is macrobiotics?" I like the simplicity of his statement. It captures the feeling I have every time I sit down to eat. Once you are eating grains and vegetables on a regular basis, you will be able to understand what Joe meant by his remark. At first, you will begin to feel better and to look younger and brighter. Your thinking and reasoning abilities will become keener. After a short while, you will notice that your taste buds have changed. When this happens, and it will happen quickly, you will stop craving food that is detrimental to your health. The body has its own wisdom, and you will naturally crave healthful food. Hard as it is to believe, sooner or later, bacon and eggs will seem foreign to you!

I want to be clear about this: Americans must change their ideas about the meaning of complete nutrition. The modern practice of eating a lot of protein, especially animal protein, leads to serious illness. There is a real crisis in the healthcare industry because health-insurance companies cannot keep up with the huge numbers of people needing medical help and hospitalization. If you accept the concept that we are what we eat and that food can ei ther make us sick or keep us well, then you must conclude that both as a nation and as individuals, we have been making the worst possible food choices for a very long time.

Grains and Vegetables

If we want good health, it is crucial that we return to a diet based on unrefined foods and complex carbohydrates. A grain or grain product and at least one vegetable dish should be eaten at every meal—including breakfast. This may take some getting used to; but after a while, if you aren't able to have a vegetable as part of your breakfast, you will really miss having it. Vegetables complete cereal grains nutritionally, and they will help you to feel more satisfied with your meals. Try to use a variety of cooking styles and a variety of vegetables, because the more you vary both, the better your health will become. Green leafy vegetables, broccoli, and cabbage are all excellent sources of calcium and vitamin C, and they contain a surprising amount of protein.

Most of my children do not like "protein dishes." Some will eat beans occasionally, most like tofu but not tempeh, and only a few of them like seitan (a wheat gluten product). Most of them do like fish, but we serve fish only a few times a month.

In spite of this, they are mostly in the top fifty percent of their grade for height and weight. Where does their protein for growth come from? The only possibility is the combination of grains and vegetables. Fruit, oil, and grain-based sweets are also a regular part of their diet, and I am sure that these foods contribute to their growth as well.

Highlights:
- Grains and/or grain products are the center-piece of a meal.
- Choose your grain first when planning a meal.
- Soft-cooked grains such as oatmeal or soft rice are best for breakfast.
- Eat brown rice often or daily.
- Grains have the ideal balance of minerals, pro-teins, and carbohydrates that our body needs for balance and proper nourishment.
- You do not need to worry about the overall proportion of grains. Just eat a comfortable, satisfying amount.
- Start off with an equal portion of grains and vegetables.

COMPLETE AND BALANCE EVERY MEAL WITH ONE OR TWO VEGETABLE DISHES.

"The greatest delight the fields and woods minister is the suggestion of an occult relation between man and the vegetable. I am not alone and unacknowl-edged. They nod to me and I to them."
— Ralph Waldo Emerson

A Matter of Balance

What do we mean by balance? In order to feel satisfied, our bodies require a certain proportion of basic nutrients. We need approximately seven times more protein than minerals. This one-to-seven ratio represents a balance or an averaging of the numbers between one and ten and is not arbitrary. It derives from the workings of the natural environment. The rotation of the earth on its axis creates a powerful energy that we call earth's force—energy that is released upward from the center of the earth. The movement of the universe also creates a powerful energy—energy that flows downward toward the center of the earth and that we call heaven's force. Heaven's force is seven times greater than earth's force. This is why, in order to escape the earth's gravity and move into outer space, a rocket needs seven thousand pounds of thrust.

Around the world and down the centuries, definitions of balance and beauty have been based on this one-to-seven ratio. For example, classical Greek statues of the fourth century B.C., the Golden Age of Greece, have heads that are approximately one-seventh the size of their bodies. That which is aesthetically beautiful and pleasing to the human eye is not arbitrary either. Rather, it is based on our innate sense of balance, a sense that comes directly from Nature.

Many things conform to the one-to-seven ratio, including the ratio of nutrients necessary to maintain human health and well-being. For example, if you eat a hard-boiled egg (concentrated protein), you will undoubtedly want to sprinkle some salt (minerals) on it. Salt improves the taste of eggs and makes them more digestible. Tofu needs soy sauce to make it tastier and easier to digest. The human body requires seven times as much carbohydrate as protein. If we eat meat, we quite naturally crave potatoes or beer or sugar—some type of carbohydrate—to balance the meat and make it digestible.

Grain is the only food that conforms to these ideal proportions. Grain contains about seven times as much protein as minerals and seven times as much carbohydrate as protein. Meat contains no carbohydrates. Therefore, meat by itself cannot completely satisfy us. Vegetables contain some carbohydrates but not in the one-to-seven proportion. Beans come closer than any food group besides grains.

Fat is a balancing agent between proteins and carbohydrates. The body has no difficulty converting fat into either protein or carbohydrate. If the body needs energy, it breaks fat down into glucose. Glucose provides the energy. Fat is converted to protein all the time. When we work out, we are converting fat into muscle protein. Conversely, protein can easily convert to fat if we eat too much protein or if we are not active.

Here's an important and little-known fact. Refined carbohydrates can produce fat in the body. This means that although many foods do not themselves contain cholesterol, they can create cholesterol. Overeating can also raise cholesterol levels. Craving or eating a lot of fat is a sign that your diet is out of balance. Fat is the nutrient that is most easily converted into protein or carbohydrate in the body. If our diet approximates the one-to-seven proportion of proteins and carbohydrates, we will not crave fat. This is why it is possible to follow a macrobiotic way of eating— which is very low in fat—and feel satisfied. Grain eating is balanced eating.

Simple and Complex Nutrients—Eat One and You Will Crave the Other

There is another element to consider when attempting to balance our diet. If we eat simple minerals, such as sodium chloride (common table salt), we will naturally begin to crave complex, or denser, protein—either animal protein or very dense vegetable protein. When we eat simple minerals, meat tastes better to us. If we eat complex animal or dairy protein, we will crave simple (refined) carbohydrates. In practical terms, this means that a hamburger won't taste right on a whole-wheat bun. The complex protein of the hamburger is not attracted to the complex carbohydrate of the whole-wheat bun. Or take the example of fish sushi. Of course, it tastes much better with white rice than with brown because, as we now understand, complex craves simple. By contrast, vegetable sushi, a simple protein, tastes better with brown rice, a complex carbohydrate.

If you eat white rice, white bread, sugar, and other simple carbohydrates like potatoes, your body will begin to crave more complex protein, usually animal and dairy foods. On the other hand, if you introduce complex minerals into your diet—in the form of unrefined white sea salt (not Celtic or gray salt, please), seaweed, and pickles—you will find yourself craving more complex carbohydrates, such as whole unrefined grains and beans and vegetables. Here's a rewarding fact of macrobiotic life. Once you are eating whole grains on a daily basis, you will naturally begin to crave food that is good for you!

Refusing vegetables

As a child, I refused to eat vegetables. Lettuce and tomato (in a sandwich) were the only exceptions. My mother was an excellent cook, but I didn't appreciate her skills. Food was a problem for me. Once a week I was permitted to have dinner out with my friends. These were the meals I liked best. I ate all the junk food my body could handle. Whether consciously or not, throughout my childhood I refused vegetables completely. I would eat my mother's vegetable soup only if she strained out the vegetables. I was that bad! In light of this confession, it strikes me as highly ironic that I have spent most of my adult life trying to persuade other people to eat their vegetables.

Within a week of incorporating brown rice into my diet, I started to enjoy vegetables. I even began to crave them. The very food I had refused to eat for so long was suddenly appetizing and desirable. Perhaps I have even caught up with those of you who were smart enough to have eaten vegetables all along. What I'm trying to convey is the fact that the process of moving from an unhealthful diet to a healthful one occurs naturally, if we follow some simple guidelines. Once we eat brown rice and vegetables on a regular basis, our cravings for unhealthful food tend to disappear.

Seaweed seduced me next. Seaweed amazed me. I remember walking into Sanae, the only macrobiotic restaurant in Boston, on a cold day in February of 1969 and ordering hiziki on impulse. The taste was new to me, neither good nor bad, but the memory of it stayed with me. The hiziki felt right in my body and I wanted to try it again. I have grown to truly love the taste of all seaweed and the way it makes me feel. My observation is that almost everyone grows to love seaweed. For some it takes time, others enjoy it immediately. Seaweed is unique, one of the more primitive foods we have. It provides a kind of nourishment and satisfaction that few other foods offer.

Perhaps it's akin to the love of raw oysters and clams that some of us develop. These are also primitive foods, but seaweed is vegetable-quality and has a wider appeal. My research has shown me that seaweed was traditionally eaten by all major cultures except those in Africa, where people ate river and lake weeds instead. In our own country, some American Indian tribes traveled great distances to harvest seaweed.

Upsetting the Balance
There are various ways in which we may upset the balance inherent in the macrobiotic diet. One way is by eating too much baked or roasted or toasted food. In essence, baking, roasting, or toasting is carbonizing. If you burn a piece of toast, what you are left with is carbon. Although carbon is a mineral common to all living things, the catch is that once we increase the amount of carbon in our diet through baking, toasting, roasting, or burning, we automatically begin to crave more complex proteins (animal and dairy food) as well as refined grains. Excess carbon throws off the body's entire mineral balance. Cravings for strong foods, such as meat, appear; feelings of guilt and despair occur, and the person to whom this is happening doesn't understand why. Too much baked or roasted or toasted food can be a recipe for disaster.

There are many tempting macrobiotic baked products available in health food stores today; so it's important to keep in mind that if you eat too many of these products, you will find it difficult to resist the lure of other unhealthful foods. Try to limit your intake of baked foods of all kinds, including bagels. It's okay to indulge yourself once in a while, but certainly not on a regular basis.

If a little is good, a lot is not

The other most common way of upsetting the balance of the macrobiotic diet is by using too much seaweed, especially kombu. Kombu is a type of kelp that is very beneficial to health. It helps lower fat and cholesterol levels, among other things. Seaweed, including kombu, is also a good source of minerals—calcium is one of them—but eating too much kombu over a long period of time can interfere with mineral absorption. To absorb minerals, we need some oil or fat in our diet, and seaweed directly affects how the body utilizes oil and fat.

People tend to think that if a little of something is good for them, then more must be even better; but often that's not true. Excess can lead to serious deficiency. In the case of seaweed, less is more—meaning less is better. Seaweed should be taken in small amounts, but people typically increase their intake over time—often dramatically. As I just mentioned, too much seaweed can interfere with the body's ability to absorb minerals. The following is what can happen if we become mineral-deficient because of an excessive intake of seaweed: in an attempt to regain its ability to absorb minerals, the body develops strong cravings for fat and protein; we begin to eat more fat and protein. Then because we feel better after eating this way, we assume it must be good for us—we must have needed more animal food. Looked at in one way, this is not an incorrect assumption. In order to overcome an imbalance, the body cries out for fat. But you can see that it would be far better not to create an imbalance at all. Be careful with the quantity of seaweed you use. It's important not to upset your body's mineral balance.

There's another problem with eating too much seaweed. One of the things the body does with fat is to convert it into sex hormones. If we decrease the body's fat content too much, in other words, if there isn't enough fat available because its absorption has been interfered with—and an overuse of seaweed and salt can do this—we invite an imbalance of sex hormones.

Highlights:
- Have at least one vegetable dish with every meal, including breakfast.
- Have a variety of vegetable dishes—well cooked, lightly cooked, pressed, pickled, and raw throughout the days and weeks.
- Grains and vegetables together provide the basis of complete and balanced nutrition.
- Do not reheat leftover vegetable dishes. They lose their refreshing and nourishing qualities and leave you unsatisfied. If they have been refrigerated, take them out in advance and let them warm up naturally.

ACTIVATE AND HARMONIZE YOUR DIGESTION WITH A SERVING OF VEGETABLE SOUP AT ONE OR TWO MEALS DAILY.

Let's take a closer look at soup. Soup conditions or relaxes the digestive system and readies it to accept the meal. As I mentioned earlier, there are basically two types of soup—savory (what one ordinarily thinks of as vegetable soup) and puréed sweet vegetable soup.

Generally, savory soups, such as miso vegetable, bean vegetable, or shoyu (natural soy sauce) vegetable broth, are taken at the beginning of the meal. Most vegetables or bean soups that we are familiar with are savory soups. Sweet vegetable soups are eaten throughout the meal. If you find this confusing, the safest approach is to eat your soup at the start of your meal.

All savory soups activate digestion. If a naturally fermented seasoning such as miso or shoyu is cooked into the soup, it will further aid the digestive process. Fermentation helps create good bacteria, yeast, and enzymes to form a healthful environment in the intestines.

All sweet vegetable soups, being mild and sweetly creamy, help to relax, harmonize, and coordinate the digestive system and its central organs—the pancreas, stomach, liver, and gallbladder. When these organs are aligned, digestion is smoother. Sweet vegetable soup does not have to be puréed although it is more effective that way.

> "An old-fashioned vegetable soup, without any enhancement, is a more powerful anti-carcinogen than any known medicine."
> —James Duke, M.D. (USDA)

More savory than sweet vegetable soup
We all need a combination of sweet and savory soups, but we need about two to three times more savory soup. Serve puréed sweet vegetable soup two to three times in a seven-to-ten-day period, and eat a variety of savory soups the rest of the time. Any vegetable soup that has either miso, shoyu, or sea salt cooked in it is a savory soup. For instance, you can turn lentil vegetable soup into miso soup by seasoning it with miso. If

you take the same soup and season it with shoyu, you create lentil-vegetable shoyu soup. Both versions qualify as savory.

Relieving Stress
Foods with a creamy texture are more relaxing and consoling, and that soothing quality has a positive effect on the digestive system. During the Great Depression, sales of ice cream skyrocketed. People had no money for anything other than the bare essentials; nevertheless, they bought ice cream. During really hard, stressful times, it seems we seek creamy foods for consolation. If you make sure you have the proper amount of sweet, creamy soup, you will have an easier time controlling the stress level in your everyday life. Stress hardens and tightens the digestive organs. Puréed soup helps them stay relaxed. Remember, if you're feeling nervous or pressured, it's important to take a few minutes to relax before sitting down to eat.

"Soup puts the heart at ease, calms down the violence of hunger, eliminates the tension of the day, and awakens and refines the appetite."
—Auguste Escoffier

Miso Soup
Miso soup has always been an important part of the macrobiotic diet. Recently, it's made its way into the mainstream—perhaps because it's so easy to prepare. Please consider restricting your intake of miso soup to what you make at home. The quality of miso paste used by restaurants is often very poor. Traditionally, it took one to two years to age and ferment miso properly. By artificially controlling temperature

and using chemical fermentation, commercial miso can be made in one week! As an added insult, commercial miso is often flavored and dyed and may even contain monosodium glutamate (MSG), an unhealthful chemical preservative and taste enhancer. Commercial miso doesn't have any of the benefits that naturally fermented miso, available in most health food stores, has.

More is not better
It's important to have one or two bowls of soup a day. One bowl is generally enough. If you feel like having a second bowl, by all means have it. If you do have a second soup, try to make it a different type of soup.

For most people however, two soups every day is too much. Eating soup with every meal is definitely a bad idea. As with many other food choices in the macrobiotic diet, more soup is not better. Too much soup, rather than strengthening digestion, will weaken it. As for quantity, a standard cup or small bowl-sized serving is adequate. Please keep in mind that a bowl of soup by itself does not qualify as a meal—even if it contains a grain. It's important to understand that soup, whether it's miso or shoyu or sweet vegetable, does not count as a complete and nutritionally balanced meal—at breakfast or at any other time.

Which brings me to my next point. For many years, macrobiotic teaching has recommended taking miso soup at breakfast. However, it's been my observation that some people are hungry all day long if they do this and, as a result, they overeat. Why? Miso soup has a powerful capacity to stimulate digestion; and when digestion is stimulated, we want to eat. I now recommend taking miso soup no more than once a day at whatever meal works best for you. Experiment. Try it for breakfast on one day, lunch on another and, on another day, for dinner. See at which time it works best for you, at which time you leave the table feeling most satisfied.

Highlights:
- There are two main types of soup: savory vegetable soup is well seasoned and mildly salty; puréed sweet vegetable soup is mildly sweet with a pleasant creamy taste.
- Soup with a savory taste activates digestion and stimulates the appetite.
- Puréed sweet vegetable soup helps relax and harmonize the digestive system. It has a calming and consoling effect.
- Have two to three times more savory than sweet soups, i.e., two to three bowls of sweet vegetable soup in a seven-to-ten-day period.

INCORPORATE A WIDE VARIETY OF FOODS INTO YOUR DIET.

Natural foods come in an endless variety of interesting combinations, tastes, and textures. If you make an effort to try new foods and new recipes, I can assure you that your taste in food will change quickly.

Greater variety in your diet will make you feel more satisfied and will provide better nutrition as well. Start by adding a few new foods each week. The biggest mistake beginners make is to find a few foods they like and eat them over and over. Although this approach might work for a while, in the end it leads to boredom and dissatisfaction. It is also nutritionally limited. As you become more familiar with natural foods, you will gain confidence in your ability to create satisfying, healthful, and exciting meals. The more new foods you add to your diet, the more your taste for natural foods will return.

I use the word "return" because I believe our taste for healthful food is natural. Years of eating unwisely sap our ability to enjoy natural foods. My proof is that young children love well-prepared natural foods on their first try. From time to time throughout the years, my children have been reluctant to invite their friends over for fear they wouldn't like our way of eating. Usually these friends enjoy the food so much, they ask for seconds. If they don't like our food the first time, they usually come around after a few more tries.

There is far more variety available in a plan-based way of eating than in the modern American diet. The key to success is to consciously increase variety over time. Now that so many supermarkets carry natural foods and organic produce, you can start your education there. Once you feel more confident, make a trip to your local health-food store.

The Healthful Foods List and Recipes section includes a sample grocery list, as well as ideas to help with familiarizing yourself with some common and delicious preparations of these foods.

Styles of Cooking
Try to use a wide variety of cooking styles when you prepare your meals. The macrobiotic repertoire is extensive. For daily use, I recommend pressure-cooking, boiling, blanching, steaming, steaming with kombu seaweed (called nishime style), soup-making, stewing, quick sautéeing with water or oil, sautéeing and simmering (kinpira style), pressing and pickling, and raw. On the Styles of Cooking list toward the back of this

book, you will find baking, broiling, dry-roasting, pan-frying, deep-frying, and tempura (batter-dipped deep-frying) food listed under Occasional Use.

When planning your meals, select foods within the following categories: whole grains, soups, vegetables, beans, sea vegetables, and beverages. Use different cooking methods from the above list. Keep in mind that it's best not to pressure-cook vegetables. Start with those cooking styles that are familiar. If possible, take macrobiotic or natural foods cooking classes. Read cookbooks to inspire and teach you.

Vegetables can be cut in various ways. Try slicing them into rounds or half-moons. You can cut the slices straight across or on the diagonal and you can vary the thickness of the slices. Different methods have subtly different effects on the flavor and appearance of whatever dish you prepare.

Vary the kinds of seasoning and condiments you use. Use different seasonings in dishes you are familiar with and take note of how just a small change in the seasoning of a dish can produce a big difference in taste. Try seasoning that same dish with a little more or less of what you normally use. The type and amount of seasoning will each bring out different aspects of flavor and can subtly alter the consistency of a dish. Some seasonings firm up a dish, so to speak, while others have a softening effect.

It's important to vary the cooking time of vegetables. Most of us could use more lightly cooked vegetables in our diet. What do I mean by a lightly cooked vegetable? It's one that makes a crunchy sound when you bite into it. The sound should be audible to someone sitting next to you. No sound means the vegetable is well cooked. Include a combination of well cooked and lightly cooked vegetable dishes weekly. Experiment with cooking times. Cook familiar dishes a little longer or for a little less time. And don't forget that raw salad is an important part of the macrobiotic diet. Have a salad at least a few times a week. In most cases, it's fine on a daily basis.

Try varying the intensity of the flame when you cook. The same dish can taste quite different depending on whether it's been cooked slowly or quickly. Many people use too much fire when cooking. It seems to be a natural tendency to turn the flame up as high as possible, whether it's needed or not. Excessive use of a high flame in your cooking may make you nervous or irritable. Use a medium flame when you want to bring something to a boil. If necessary, you can always turn it up at the end of cooking. You will feel calmer and steadier as a result.

Vary the combination of dishes you use in meals. Change just one dish and you have added a new meal to your repertoire. And vary the combination of vegetables, grains, beans, and seasonings you use in your dishes.

Cook your food a little longer in the winter for a warming, energizing effect. Cooking food a bit less in the summer will produce a cooling and relaxing effect.

Try to create a variety of color, taste, and consistency in your meals. Variety means using many different ingredients from each of the different categories, changing the method of preparation and changing the combinations of food. Imagine what the meal will look like on the plate, imagine how it will taste. Remember that variety creates interest. Try to surprise your family and friends. Keep them guessing. They are sure to enjoy and appreciate your efforts.

Suggestions for Planning Meals

First considerations

- Grains and vegetables together form the basis of complete and balanced nutrition.
- All food has protein. You do not need to make a special effort to increase protein in your diet. It is nearly impossible to become protein-deficient.
- If you feel that you are craving protein, increase beans, tofu, tempeh, seitan, and possibly add fish.
- A variety of vegetable foods provides the most abundant and well-balanced nutrition available: minerals including calcium, potassium, proteins, carbohydrates, fats including omega-3, and vitamins including vitamin C. Vitamin D comes from exposing your skin to the sun.
- Beans may be included in the same meal or even the same dish as fish.
- Seitan, a wheat gluten product, may be cooked with grains or beans.

When planning your daily meals, try to follow the order below

- Always decide on the grain or grain product first.
- Then choose the vegetable dish and/or dishes that complement and harmonize the grain.
- Next, decide on the soup to further complete the meal.
- Last, supplement with foods from the other categories, specifically beans, sea vegetables,

seeds, nuts, fish, fruit, snacks, desserts, sweets, and beverages, if you choose.

- Use these guidelines whether you are eating at home or out.

Questions to ask when planning every meal

- What grains or grain products do I want?
- What vegetable dishes do I want?
- Will they be freshly prepared or leftover?

Questions to ask every day

- What soup will I have today?
- Am I including brown rice in one of my meals today?
- What beans and/or bean products shall I have today?
- Am I including a variety of well cooked, lightly cooked (meaning bright, colorful and crunchy), and raw vegetable dishes?

Questions to ask when planning your weekly menu

- Am I incorporating sea vegetables into my diet?
- Shall I have fish this week?
- What desserts and snacks shall I have?
- Am I getting enough variety in the other categories, including seeds, nuts, fish, fruit, mild natural sweets, and beverages?
- Are my meals appealing, tasty, colorful, and satisfying?

- Have I remembered to incorporate leftovers to
  save time on cooking?

ORDER OF PLANNING MEALS

	MODERN DIET	MACROBIOTIC DIET
1. Principal Foods, the centerpiece of every meal	**Protein:** Meat, poultry, eggs, cheese, or fish; For vegetarians: Beans, soy products, textured soy protein, etc.	**Grains or Grain Products:** Brown rice, barley, millet, polenta, pasta, oatmeal, couscous, whole wheat bread, etc.
2. Main Secondary Foods, they complete, balance, and harmonize every meal	**Starch:** Potatoes, pasta, bread, white rice, or other refined grains	**Vegetables:** Well cooked, lightly cooked, pressed salad, pickles, raw salad
3. Soup with 1 or 2 meals a day	Infrequent	Miso, vegetable, lentil, puréed squash, etc.
4. Other Foods throughout the week	Salad, vegetables, fruits, snacks and sweets, dessert, or beverages	Beans, seeds, nuts, fish, fruit, snacks, dessert, beverages
5. Essence of a Meal	Protein, starch, and beverage	Grain, vegetable, and soup
6. Typical Meals	Meat, potatoes and coffee Pizza and soda Pizza and beer Hamburger, fries, and soda Omelet, fries, toast, and coffee	Brown rice, steamed kale or collards, and bancha twig tea Couscous, sautéed onion and broccoli, and miso soup Steamed tofu sandwich on whole- wheat bread with tahini and sauerkraut and apple juice Pasta, vegetables, and tea, spring water, or beer Polenta, broccoli rabe, red snapper, and wine

Highlights:

- Create variety by varying the ingredients in each of the categories, changing the method of preparation and the combination of foods in the dishes you create.
- Try not to settle on a few dishes and combinations and then continually repeat them.
- Variety ensures the most balanced nutrition and helps you feel more satisfied.
- All foods contain protein. The vegetable protein in grains, beans, and vegetables is superior to animal protein for health.

BUY THE HIGHEST-QUALITY ORGANICALLY GROWN, UNREFINED, NON-GMO, AND NATURALLY PROCESSED FOODS.

High-quality organic food tastes better. It's more nourishing and strengthening to your health. Many people are willing to buy expensive cars, clothes, and houses, but when it comes to buying food they won't spend the extra money for the best quality. Please, don't save money on your food. Try to buy mostly organically grown food, in particular, staples like daily-use vegetables and grains, miso, sea vegetables, shoyu, ume and brown rice vinegars and umeboshi plums etc., even if you have to travel or mail-order to do it. What is not available, you can certainly supplement with commercially grown food. If most of your food is organically grown, then some unrefined and commercially produced food is not going to harm you and you will enjoy the benefits of increased variety.

That said, it's vital to remember that quality can be adjusted up or down. Here's an example of what I mean: If you think Diet (Content and Quality) is more important than Eating Habits (Format) and you want to eat organically grown, pressure-cooked short or medium grain brown rice, but it's not available to you at that moment, then what do you do? Well, many people think if they can't practice perfectly, if they can't have the best food all the time, then they're not good macrobiotics. So they abandon the diet temporarily and proceed to make terrible choices. This is a pretty common response, particularly when traveling. However, if you want to eat well, you can eat well under any circumstances. If you have a health problem, the best thing to do is prepare ahead so you don't get stuck. An understanding of the controlling factors of macrobiotic practice and how to adapt to difficult circumstances is very important.

Adjusting quality
Let me explain what I mean when I say that quality can be adjusted up or down. Despite what you might think, white rice and commercially made pasta qualify as a grain and grain product. Steamed vegetables without butter are still vegetables. You can order vegan vegetable soup. Will it be macrobiotic quality? No, not exactly. It may be made with potatoes or tomatoes or both but it's still vegetable soup. Remember that as long as you stick to the Format, you will be moving in the direction of health. To tell if you are becoming lax about the Format, watch for danger signals such as reading or watching TV at the table, eating or snacking while standing, not chewing thoroughly, rushing

through meals, not allowing three hours between eating and sleeping and so on. If these things begin to happen and you are not alert to them, it's only a matter of time before you create an imbalance, and imbalances tend to perpetuate themselves. So long as you concentrate on the Format of Meals (Eating Habits), over time your diet will become more and more healthful. You will come to understand intuitively what you need to improve and maintain good health. But if you focus on Diet (Content and Quality of Meals), then automatically you will begin thinking in terms of good and bad, right and wrong, calcium and protein, etc., and when we think this way we get off track. It's very easy to fall into this sort of thinking. It's the way we've been taught, and modern education, being so powerful, is hard to overcome.

Our goal is simply this: to have good digestion, good absorption, and good circulation. After all, what is the difference between being young and being old? The answer is good digestion, good absorption, and good circulation. If the food that enters the body can be digested and absorbed and the excess evacuated easily and if the blood can circulate, then we can cure ourselves of anything. We can reverse the effects of illness and unnatural aging, if we practice accurately. We can even wind back our biological clock and become much younger than our biological age.

Vegetarian?
We've found that many restaurants use chicken stock in so-called vegetarian dishes. It is better not to make assumptions. If you're eating away from home, it is best to ask whether

meat, poultry, or chicken stock were used in the preparation of the food.

Highlights:
- High-quality food tastes better.
- It's more nourishing and strengthening to your health.
- Quality can be adjusted up or down.
- Buy organically grown food as much as possible. Supplement with commercially grown food when the full variety of organic food is unavailable.
- Make sure to choose non-GMO foods.

LIFESTYLE:
APPROACH TO HEALTH

MAKE YOUR DAILY LIFE ACTIVE

WALK OUTSIDE FOR 30 MINUTES EVERY DAY. LIFE-RELATED EXERCISE PROVIDES THE MOST BENEFIT FOR LASTING HEALTH.
I want to encourage you to make your daily life as active as you can by incorporating what I call universal exercise. Universal exercise means life-related exercise—activities directly connected to life. These are the activities that provide the most benefit and balance for all of us.

When do you think people were generally healthier—in the past when they led physically active daily lives, or today when they are so exercise-conscious? I always ask this question in seminars and the audience almost always responds: "In the past."

Healthy people rarely think about exercise. Their lives are so active that there's no need. They play; they enjoy and challenge themselves; they may garden, do home repairs, dance, or engage in sports. In other words, they are active but they are not formally exercising. We've been educated to think we need structured exercise. We don't. What we need is to move our bodies, to play, to enjoy ourselves physically, to challenge and stimulate ourselves. Structured exercise has a kind of hardness and rigidity about it; play has a soft and flexible quality.

Here's an analogy I like. Who is healthier—the person who eats a healthful diet or the person who eats an inadequate diet and takes supplements? My point is that since healthy people are clearly getting all the nourishment they need from their diet, the idea of taking supplements never occurs to them.

Let's apply this observation to exercise. Structured exercise is nothing more than a supplement for those people who have inadequate daily activity. In order to feel well, those who lead sedentary lives have to compensate with some kind of regular program of exercise.

Exercise versus play

Healthy children never think about exercise until they go to school where they are taught that they need to exercise. Before that they simply played and were healthy and happy. Children lose their energy only when they're told to do something they don't want to do, such as cleaning their rooms. A child's natural need to move is changing now because of poor diet. It's not natural for children to want to sit around all day and watch television. My children enjoy television but they know it's self-limiting. After a while they are always running off to do something else. Only on rare occasions do I have to say "That's enough TV."

The best exercise for your health is the exercise that human beings were designed to do, exercise that doesn't require machinery, gyms, or classes. Like the air we breathe, it's free of charge. I refer to walking. Walking outside at a comfortable pace with an unforced stride is the best exercise on the planet.

Don't worry about cardiovascular rates and, please, don't engage in "power walking." The value of walking comes from the rhythmic movement—not the pace. A somewhat brisk half-hour walk every day (or two fifteen-minute ones) will keep the body fit and the spirits high. Walking increases flexibility and improves digestion, energy, and cardiovascular health. It strengthens the bones and helps clear the mind and balance the nervous system. Walking is the ideal activity for everyone. It is the brown rice of physical activity, so to speak.

It's best not to think of walking as "exercise" per se. You can think of it as a way to get from point A to point B, if you like; you can think of it as a period of time to clear your mind and let your thoughts come. The more open your mind is when you walk, the more benefit you will receive. The people who get the least out of walking are the ones who are trying to accomplish something, such as getting their heart rate up. Why? When we have an agenda, the mind closes to other possibilities. Take children as your model. Children have the best activity; they play and enjoy themselves. They don't think they're exercising or getting healthy. As long as they're playing and enjoying themselves, their minds are open.

If strenuous exercise were the panacea it is said to be, then professional athletes would be among the healthiest people in the world. Yet this is not the case. Many, perhaps even a majority, of them suffer from serious chronic injuries and other health problems. Many die young. Modern nutritional thinking says that large amounts of animal food are necessary for building stamina and keeping a competitive edge. As a result, the diet of athletes is usually high in meat, dairy products, and refined carbohydrates. Athletes are given to believe that their health will not suffer since participation in strenuous sports compensates for dietary excess. Now, you don't have to be a genius to understand that if you eat excessively, your body will suffer the effects regardless of how much you exercise. It's a matter of common sense.

Not too long ago, I saw the results of a research study on the immune system of professional athletes as compared to that of the average person. According to this study, the immune system of the professional athlete is weaker than that of the average person. Apparently, professional athletes are more likely to come down with colds than are those who don't compete professionally. When the body is overworked, immunity is impaired. Pushing the body beyond its natural limits in any way is not a healthful thing to do.

"The sovereign invigorator of the body is exercise, and of all exercises walking is the best."
—Thomas Jefferson

Walking and balance
It's not necessary to walk briskly for a full half-hour at one time. Two fifteen-minute walks are also effective. Keep in mind that the benefits of walking come from the balancing effect of rhythmic movement on the body. We derive the greatest benefits from walking when our arms are free to swing like a pendulum. The alternating movement of arms and legs has a balancing effect on the body as a whole, and on its functions as well. To be specific, this is what happens: both parts of the digestive system, the ascending and the descending

colon, coordinate with each other; the left lung and the right lung do the same. Both branches of the autonomic nervous system—that part of the overall nervous system that regulates breathing, digestion, and, in fact, all of the body's automatic functions—are coordinated and brought into balance.

At the same time, walking helps balance the mind. When you feel anxious or worried, try taking a walk. After a short time, you will find yourself thinking more clearly and, in general, feeling better. If you are depressed, taking a walk will refresh your spirits. If you are overtired, a walk will renew your energy. If you have too much energy, a walk will settle you down.

> "Today I have grown taller from walking with trees."
>
> —Karl Baker

Walk outdoors
Walking outdoors is far more beneficial than walking indoors. We need to be outside for one simple but compelling reason. Nature has the best circulation. Anything we do outdoors helps our circulation more than anything done inside. A walk outside in pleasant surroundings, in the woods or in a park, for example, amid grass and trees, is ideal; but even a walk on a busy city street is better than walking inside on a treadmill or track. When you walk, the quality of the air you take in is important and, as a rule, outdoor air is less polluted than indoor air. With this in mind, try to keep your home or office well ventilated. Open your windows.

Do healthy people exercise?

Let's consider an earlier statement of mine: Healthy people rarely think about exercising. The fact is that the most valuable exercise occurs as we go about living our daily lives. When we walk, shop, clean, or do other things around the house, we are exercising without really thinking about it. And when we are active while doing what we enjoy—whether it's dancing, tennis, martial arts, swimming, mountain-climbing, or biking—we are exercising without having to force ourselves. It's important to find activities that are satisfying, challenging, and stimulating. The thought should not be "I have to do this, it's good for me," but rather "I can't wait to get out there and do this." It's simply common sense that if you engage in activities you enjoy, you will keep on doing them and never think of them as "exercise." I want to be very clear about this. I am not saying don't exercise. What I'm saying is this: Make your life active. Do whatever stimulates and challenges you. If you think it's "good" for you, don't do it.

Again, take healthy children as a model. Observe them. See how they always try to challenge and stimulate themselves. When they've had enough of something, they move on to something else.

Many people find daily exercise combined with a healthful diet to be the easiest Strengthening Health recommendation to follow. Walking is an enjoyable way to keep physically fit. If you are not already in the habit of walking, you will be surprised by the deep sense of well-being that a daily walk gives.

"All truly great thoughts are conceived by walking."
—Friedrich Nietzsche

A Barometer

If our exercise is appropriate, our appetite for healthful food will be enhanced. Appropriate exercise helps us eat less and feel more satisfied. We can tell that our exercise is inappropriate if our craving for rich food and sweets increases, if we overeat but feel less satisfied.

Cleaning

In more traditional times, even as recently as fifty years ago, cleaning was valued in proportion to its benefits. Cleanliness, of both person and surroundings, was said to be next in importance to godliness. Like walking, the benefits of cleaning are universal—unless you have an attitude about it! We feel better physically and mentally when we clean. Cleaning clears the mind as it activates the body. It helps harmonize and balance our condition. Try it and you'll see.

Obesity in children

Obesity is a major problem in the United States. Approximately two out of three adults are overweight and more than one in six children are overweight or obese. "Morbidly obese" is the term used to define that degree of obesity that is considered life-threatening. There are so many obese children that even the government has been forced to take notice. Obesity in children is the cause of the current epidemic of Childhood Onset Diabetes. Obesity starts with diet. Children who are fed too many high-fat foods and sweets are less inclined to run around and play because their young bodies are too busy trying to metabolize all the excess. These children are most comfortable slumped in front of a TV set or computer for hours at a time.

Many of my children's friends are not from macrobiotic families, so at our birthday parties we usually serve ice cream and other sugared foods to make their friends feel comfortable. Of course, there are always plenty of macrobiotic goodies as well. Over the past decade, I've noticed that often these children hardly touch the cake and ice cream, although my children usually eat their fair share. My explanation of this seemingly odd behavior is that these children don't find party foods to be anything special. These foods are special for my children because they don't have them very often. For their friends, however, cake and ice cream are actually everyday foods. The result is an ever-increasing rate of obesity among children.

A healthful diet creates a natural craving for activity. It's a kind of chain reaction. We need a good diet in order to be active. If we are active and if we are satisfied with our food, chances are we won't find ourselves overeating.

War and Nutrition

If we use history as a guide, we can see the effects of the decline in nutrition and activity levels by analyzing the health of the soldiers who fought in various wars. Roman soldiers were hired mercenaries. They were paid in grain, primarily an ancient type of barley, and this grain was their principal source of nutrition. Fueled by a grain-based diet, Roman soldiers conquered almost half the world. Roman generals maintained a strict daily regimen that kept their legions fit for the task of conquering strong foes, sometimes armies far larger than their own. It was not unusual for a legion to march twenty-five to thirty miles a day, each man carrying full weaponry and daily food supplies on his back. The fall of the Roman Empire followed on the heels of widespread changes in eating habits and daily activity. The Roman Legionnaires, by eating the foods of the lands they had conquered and occupied, grew lazy and gluttonous, often gorging themselves until they vomited. Banquets, at which huge amounts of food were consumed, became a daily feature of life. A downfall was inevitable.

Autopsies of young soldiers who died in action in the Korean War revealed badly clogged arteries and signs of advanced cardiovascular disease. The medical community was shocked. The question asked was whether the government's policy of feeding soldiers a high-protein, high-meat diet had caused the disease. Autopsies of soldiers who died in the Vietnam War presented similar findings. In light of the evidence, it's difficult to understand why the government took so long to change its food recommendations.

Highlights:
- Walk outside to get the maximum benefit. Walking outside aligns you with the natural environment. Contact with the earth, exposure to trees and grass and to the natural circulation of air are crucial to good health.
- Walking is not exercise. It is natural movement. It creates harmony between body and mind, improves circulation and digestion, and increases flexibility and bone strength.
- Walk once a day for a minimum of 30 minutes or twice a day for 15 minutes. A natural, comfortable stride is recommended.
- Imitate children and try to play rather than exercise.

- Life-related activities such as cleaning, gardening, dancing, etc. provide the most benefits.

GIVE YOURSELF A DAILY BODY RUB.

Gently rub your entire body with a hot, damp cotton washcloth for ten to fifteen minutes every morning and/ or night. Do the rub before or after your bath or shower, but do it separately from either. The body rub is the secret of the fountain of youth. In effect, it winds back the body's biological clock. If you do a daily body rub and if you chew your food thoroughly, day by day you will become younger in body and mind.

The body rub is one of the world's best beauty treatments. People come to me for counseling with a variety of skin problems—brown liver spots, white patches, blemishes, and skin that is loose, dry, or sagging. Often they blame these conditions on age, but I believe they have unhealthy skin because they don't know how to care for themselves.

Within a few months, sometimes as little as a few weeks, these blemishes begin to disappear. Beautiful new and younger-looking skin comes shining through. Of course, your progress depends on what you eat and how well and faithfully you do the body rub. Everyone wants to look younger and healthier. Billions of dollars are spent every year on beauty creams, remedies, and treatments, most of which don't work. The body rub is free and it does work.

New skin in 28 days

The skin completely renews itself every twenty-eight days. In essence, your skin is no more than a month old at any given moment. Cells in the skin are continuously dying and replacing themselves. We can renew our skin in a healthy or unhealthy way. How the skin renews itself depends on what we have been eating over the previous days, weeks, and months. One of the benefits of eating well is that fresh blood is drawn continuously to the surface areas of the body, stimulating the skin. If we eat healthful foods and do the body rub, we can nourish our skin on a daily basis and, as a result, our skin will become younger-looking and more beautiful. Once past puberty, people of all ages can benefit from the body rub. Healthy skin is slightly shiny and moist. If your skin is healthy, your entire body perspires lightly and easily. Such skin is smooth, soft to the touch, and resilient. If you push or pull it, it bounces back energetically. Healthy skin looks fresh without the aid of creams and moisturizers and is free of blemishes and pimples. The skin is an excellent barometer of overall health. I always use skin diagnosis in counseling. It tells me about the client's diet, past health problems, and ability to maintain good health in the future.

Most of us take our skin for granted. We all want skin that looks young and healthy, yet few of us give a thought to the skin's function. Skin is our largest organ, containing oil, sweat glands, blood vessels, nerve cells, and immune cells. It has innumerable functions. It protects us from the environment, helps to keep us warm and to cool us down, produces Vitamin D, excretes toxins, and, most importantly, keeps us in one piece!

The skin is our largest organ
The skin is a large, hard-working organ, and one of its more significant jobs is to discharge toxins from our bodies.

However, certain foods clog our skin—fatty meat, dairy products, tropical fruit, sugar, eggs, chicken, baked flour products, etc. Clogged skin means that moisture and oil cannot pass through the pores. If we eat the above-mentioned foods on a daily basis, our skin becomes dry. Most people think that dry skin is caused by a lack of oil, so they turn to the common remedy for dry skin—moisturizer. Applying such a remedy will temporarily moisten the skin, but then what happens? Where does the moisturizer go? It is absorbed into the fat layer of the skin, further clogging it, especially if the moisturizer is petroleum-based, like mineral oil and such saturated-fat products as coconut or palm oil.

The skin's tiny capillaries are connected to the body's large main arteries and veins through a vast network of blood vessels of ever-increasing size. It stands to reason that if these capillaries become clogged, the functioning of the circulatory system will be adversely affected. If the skin becomes so clogged that it can no longer discharge oil or moisture, then the excess fat and fluid go back into circulation through the blood vessels, looking, so to speak, for another exit. Over time, circulation will become sluggish, often to the point of putting a strain on the heart.

To help understand this process dynamically, it's useful to look at the mechanism of an event that occurs all too often in our daily lives—the traffic jam. A traffic jam on one road often clogs traffic on other nearby roads. It takes only one backed-up highway exit to slow the flow of traffic and overload the entire system. Most of us have experienced, to our discomfort, what happens on a late Sunday afternoon in the summer when several exits are blocked by traffic.

Nervous System, Immune System, and Meridians
There are peripheral nerve cells in the skin that govern sensitivity and sensory perception. Since the peripheral nerve cells also send messages to the central nervous system, they influence our emotions as well. In fact, the body's entire system of nerves is affected by the condition of the skin. Imbalances in the skin affect how we respond to heat, cold, touch, pressure, and vibrations. Depending on the condition of our skin, we may become over- or under-sensitive to any of the above.

The skin also contains lymphocytes, cells that are an important part of the immune system. Lymphocytes protect against viruses, bacteria, and parasites. When the skin is clogged, its ability to provide immunity is weakened.

Acupuncture meridians
Acupuncture meridians run under the skin and are connected to the body's internal organs. Meridians are not vessels or containers. They are energy streams, somewhat analogous to mountain streams, and, as such, they have precise paths. Meridians nourish the organs and allow them to discharge excess pressure. They help the internal organs regulate themselves and adjust to the environment. Although Western science does not acknowledge the existence of meridians, they have been known and used for thousands of years in the Far East. The ancient arts of acupuncture and shiatsu massage are based on and use the extensive system of meridian points.

I use meridian diagnosis extensively. It is one of my main methods for assessing someone's state of health. Meridian diagnosis gives me more information about the functioning of the body's organs and systems than any other aspect of traditional Far Eastern diagnosis. It allows me to determine how well or poorly the body's energy is flowing along its meridians. The quality of energy flow is what tells me how the corresponding organ is functioning. The meridians actually become clogged as fatty deposits collect under the skin and as organ function weakens. When the organs are not able to adjust, they lose their ability to maintain a healthy condition. They are either losing energy or building up excess pressure.

The Pressure Valve

The skin is the body's largest organ; it is also the body's largest opening. The skin functions as a kind of pressure valve. There are many ways to release pressure. Talking, writing, physical activity, urination, bowel elimination, menstruation, and sex are just some of them. Obviously, when the skin is clogged, it cannot release pressure smoothly or easily. One of the criteria of healthy skin is that its pores can open at will to release excess pressure from the body—in the same way that they open to release excess heat from the body. Our skin continually interacts with the environment in an attempt to keep the body's temperature and pressure balanced between the internal and external environments.

The body rub helps the skin function more efficiently. Clogged skin loses its ability to release internal pressure, leaving us much more adversely affected by stress. Once the skin is no longer clogged, we can release fluids and toxins the way Nature intended—by perspiring freely over our entire body. It's a commonly held belief that excess energy can be released only through exercise and activity. Not true. We all know people who talk more than seems appropriate.

What is not understood is that excessive talking is somewhat involuntary. It's the body's way of trying to rid itself of excess energy and stress. However, if the skin is open, internal pressure is released continuously. Once you are doing the body rub every day, you will be amazed at how much calmer you are and how much better you feel.

The Kidneys, Intestines, Lungs, and Liver

The kidneys are our main excretory organs. They work together with the intestines to eliminate excess from the body. The liver aids this process by detoxifying the blood. The body's normal way of discharging excess is through urination and bowel elimination. As long as the kidneys, intestines, and liver are functioning efficiently, the body will not send excess to the skin. But if these organs become tired, sluggish, or stagnated, the body's only choice is to send that excess to the surface—that is, to the skin or possibly to the lungs—for discharge.

One of the great benefits of the body rub is that it takes some of the strain off the kidneys, intestines, lungs, and liver. By helping to clean the body, the body rub gives those organs a chance to rest and repair so they can function more easily and efficiently. It is vitally important to concentrate on the health of your skin. If the skin is unable to aid in the elimination of toxins and if the kidneys, intestines, and liver are clogged and sluggish, the body has no choice but to store the excess waste, which then increases the strain on your health.

Perspiration

If you don't perspire easily, this may be an indication that your skin is dry and clogged. Perspiration is natural. Many of us perspire only from certain parts of the body, like the armpits or the forehead. If your skin is functioning properly, you should perspire from your entire body. When, for instance, you take a sauna, your pores should open easily. You should soon be covered in perspiration from head to toe. After the body rub becomes part of your daily routine, your skin will open and you will perspire freely, releasing those fluids and toxins that have been trapped inside.

Doing the Body Rub—Gently Rub, not Scrub
I have explained the dynamics of the skin's structure and function in some detail in order to help you understand the importance of the health practice that I call the body rub. The body rub is deeply cleansing to the skin. It draws out the fat that has been collecting beneath the surface and clogging your pores. A word of warning: if your skin looks and feels drier at first than it did before you began doing the body rub, take heart. This is good news. It's proof that you are doing the body rub accurately. Fat must gather under the surface of the skin before it can be discharged, and as it gathers, the skin becomes drier. I have one client who characterized the skin on her arms and legs as reptilian during the first month. Please, be patient and you will see your skin improve steadily from this point on, as she did.

The body rub is easy to do and brings immediate gratification. Some of my clients call it their morning cup of coffee—the ones who do it before bedtime report an improvement in their sleep. The body rub is easy to do. Fill your bathroom sink with the hottest tap water possible—though not scalding. The washcloth should be one hundred percent cotton, preferably unbleached or white. Fold it in half once and then in half again, making four layers. Dip the cloth in the hot water and then squeeze out the excess. The cloth should be damp but not dripping. Re-dip it in the hot water as often as necessary. Rub your skin in a back-and-forth motion, gently and systematically. A useful image is that of the tide coming in and going out. Progress in an orderly way over your entire body. You can work from the face down to the feet or from the extremities in toward the center (just below the navel).

The areas of importance are as follows:
1. Hands, wrists, fingers (and between the fingers), feet (tops and bottoms), ankles, toes (and between the toes)
2. Face and neck
3. Armpits and groin
4. Centerline of the body, from top of neck to pubic bone; chest and abdominal areas
5. Bottom of rib cage from right to left.
6. Back, including coccyx (tailbone) and sacrum
7. Elbows and knees
8. All other areas of body

If you are pressed for time, do steps 1 and 2 or 1, 2, and 3.

Do not attempt to redden your skin by using a lot of pressure. Use only the weight of your hand without pressing. Keep in mind that this is a rub and not a scrub. Your back-and-forth movement should be vigorous but gentle; light yet not too light. If there are parts of the skin that don't turn red, don't worry, just spend a bit more time on them. Eventually, when the overall condition of your skin improves and your circulation is responding to the treatment, your skin will redden quickly.

A word of caution: Many people have very delicate, weak skin. If your skin is thin and weak and you apply too much pressure, you can literally rub your skin off. You can think of the scabs that result as your battle scars! If you are very gentle in the beginning, your skin will become stronger more quickly. The initial process is similar to starting an exercise program. Begin slowly and build up gradually for the best results. Please be very careful when doing your face, especially the forehead and bridge of the nose. The skin along the spine is also exceptionally sensitive.

Keep Your Bath or Shower Separate

When you do the body rub, please do it separately from your bath or shower. Do it right before or right after. If you remain under the shower or in the tub water when doing the rub, you will lose too many vital minerals. Hot steam relaxes the body, but since steam has the capacity to draw out minerals, too much steam can be dangerous. Five to seven minutes is safe.

I recommend two methods for keeping warm if you become chilled while doing the rub, usually in winter. One is to fill the tub with hot water to just below your ankles. Then sit on the edge of the tub and proceed with the rub. The second method, the one I prefer, is to start with a very short hot shower, then turn the water off and do the rub. This allows the steam and heat from the shower to keep you warm. The bathroom will have begun to cool down by the time you are through with the rub, at which point you can finish with another very short hot shower.

Other Benefits

Another benefit of the daily body rub is that it encourages you to become more open and accepting of your body. If you really dislike doing the rub, one possibility is that you are uncomfortable with your body. In time, if you do the rub on a daily basis, your self-image will improve. You will learn to appreciate your uniqueness and you will grow to genuinely care for and respect your body. If you spend a little extra time on areas you particularly don't like, your self-image will change more quickly. Done regularly, the body rub will improve every aspect of your physical, emotional, and mental health.

A word of caution: using a loofah or dry brush is not the same practice as the body rub. The purpose of the rub is to coax the pores of the skin to open in order to draw out stored fats and toxins. If you combine hot, damp heat with the softness of a wash cloth, you can easily achieve your goal. A loofa, however, even if damp, will only impede your progress. Yes, it can remove the dead outer skin, but its very coarseness causes the pores of the living skin to close tightly, thus sealing in those fats and toxins. A dry brush may be very effective for abrading dead skin and tightening your pores, but by using one you will accomplish exactly the opposite of what you want. The body rub takes longer, but it is much more effective if your goal is to create healthy, resilient skin.

I have spent years trying to determine the best way to do the body rub, and my conclusion is that strong pressure is not as effective as light pressure. As I said earlier, the body rub is a rub, not a scrub. Light pressure applied by the natural weight of the hand is what best stimulates the circulation of energy and the opening of the pores of the skin. Once the pores can open easily, they can also close easily, and it is this easy opening and closing in response to both internal and external environments that is one of the hallmarks of resilient skin. If you do a daily body rub with a damp cloth and light pressure, you will discover this for yourself.

When you eat well and do the rub, in effect what you are doing is to draw a continuous supply of fresh blood to any given area. As for the face, one of the effects of improved circulation is the reduction and possible elimination of fine lines and wrinkles. Also, the rub improves muscle tone as well as skin texture, so that when the facial muscles are strengthened, wrinkles tend to fade or vanish.

If you've eaten a lot of cheese and other fatty and baked foods in your life, you no doubt have deposits of cellulite in your legs, hips, and buttocks. Some of my clients tell me that these parts of their bodies literally look like cottage cheese! The body rub will help break down these deposits and allow them to leave your system. Of course, if you continue to eat foods that cause cellulite, you will find yourself in an endless cycle of frustration. Now that you know the cause of cellulite, the next time you are tempted to eat cheese, just picture where it will end up. Maybe that will help you resist the temptation.

If you have very rough, red skin and feel you have to use a moisturizer, use it sparingly before going to sleep. Please don't use it in the morning. Just do the body rub. After a while, even very rough, dry skin will soften and regenerate. Except for extreme cases of very dry skin, it is unnecessary and hinders rather than helps. If used habitually, even the best-quality moisturizer can clog the skin. If you must use a moisturizer, select one made with liquid vegetable oil, such as sesame or olive; avoid any oil that becomes solid at room temperature, such as coconut oil.

Highlights:
- Use a medium-weight cotton washcloth. Fold it in half twice.
- Organic cotton is best.
- Fill your sink with hot water, dip the cloth, and wring it out. Re-dip the cloth frequently to keep it hot and fresh.
- Rub gently in a back-and-forth motion. Do not rub in circles.
- Rub gently; don't scrub. Gentle pressure yields better results.
- Do the rub separately from your bath or shower.
- The purpose of the rub is to open your pores and draw out fats and toxins. This will allow your skin to breathe naturally.
- Years of animal and dairy food, fruits, sweets, baked and fatty food clog the skin and prevent it from breathing naturally.
- The skin needs to breathe freely just as the lungs do.

Doing the body rub results in:
- An increase in the circulation of blood, lymph, and energy that will improve the nutrition,

oxygen flow, stimulation, and health of all your organs.

- Better energy all day after a morning rub and deeper sleep after an evening rub.
- More effective release of stored toxins.
- Improved immunity to disease.
- Clearer thinking, keener memory, and more optimistic outlook.
- Improved self-image.
- Increased sensual awareness.

CULTIVATE AND TAKE TIME FOR HOBBIES.

Hobbies are very, very important for good health. Yet these days how many of us have a hobby? Not many, I suspect. Hobby is a rather old-fashioned word, so I'm often asked what I mean when I use it. To me, a hobby is something that brings an aspect of completion or fullness or balance to our lives, something we do for enjoyment—a favorite activity (not passivity)—but not what we do day to day for a living.

> "To insure good health: eat lightly, breathe deeply, live moderately."
>
> —William Londen

Let me give you an example from an older time. The samurai of Japan were professional warriors, rigorously trained in the martial arts, who spent their lives fighting. To make sure their development wasn't overly one-sided, they also studied tea ceremony or poetry or brush painting, something very different, very highly refined, in order to make balance.

Now let me give you an example from modern life. I ask, "Do you have a hobby?" You answer, "Yes, reading." But if your job is mental, reading doesn't meet my definition of a hobby. A hobby has to be different from work, something that brings polarity and interest to your life.

I like this example: years ago, in *Science News*, I came across a piece about a scientist with very interesting ideas. What struck me was the fact that a couple of times a week he and his brother got together and played guitar and sang just for the fun of it. His work was technical, highly skilled, demanding and precise. His hobby released him, balanced his work. In my view, the reason he had such interesting ideas was because he spent his free time doing something he enjoyed that was very different from his work.

> "Dare to err and dare to dream. Deep meaning often lies in childish play."
> —Johann Friedrich von Schiller

Hobbies are a kind of self-reflection, a way of maintaining balance, a way to develop different sides of our nature. They are for our enjoyment, pleasure, and satisfaction. My advice is, if you don't have a hobby, choose anything you think you might enjoy. If you find you don't like it, try something else. Often clients will tell me they don't have time for a hobby. My answer is always the same: "You don't *not* have time for a hobby, because a hobby will enrich your life. Your practice and your health will improve if you have a hobby." Everything needs polarity. We add chopped parsley to sweet vegetable soup. The garnish brings the soup to life. The garnish is the hobby, in a manner of speaking.

Highlights:
- Hobbies make balance for the more structured and pressured areas of life.
- Hobbies help relieve stress and promote physical and mental flexibility.
- Have fun with your hobbies.

CREATE A MORE NATURAL ENVIRONMENT

Recharging station

What is a home? In the macrobiotic way of thinking, home is a recharging station, a place to relax, return to balance, and enrich life. Therefore, we must create the healthiest environment we can so that we are nourished rather than depleted by our surroundings. The more natural the environment around us, the brighter, more refreshed and positive we feel. Then, automatically, we make better choices in all the other areas of life.

Let's say you go on a picnic. The food tastes especially delicious and you sleep more soundly that night. Why? You're out of doors in the country with congenial company, the air is fresh, and usually you engage in some sort of physical activity. All this contributes to improved circulation. Whatever you do that improves your circulation creates a healthier appetite and a deeper, more restful night's sleep.

The direction modern life is taking is well beyond our control, but there are steps we can take that will reverse many of its worst effects. Most of us worry about those things over which we have no control, yet ignore those things we can change, things we can do every day to improve our lives. We have a choice. We can take time for our meals of grains and vegetables, stick to our daily schedule, walk, do the body rub, and surround ourselves with green plants and natural materials, on our person and in our home. Each of the first five steps, if done regularly, strengthens the effect of the others. Together, the first five steps form the essence of good health. Whether we apply these principles to the life of one person, to a family, to a community, or to a society, east, west, north, or south, they work. They are simple; they are unique. They worked in the past, they work today, and they will work in the future. Why? Because they are based on the common sense of our ancestors but adapted to modern life.

SURROUND YOURSELF WITH GREEN PLANTS.

There was a time, not so long ago, when houseplants were considered merely decorative. Walking into a house or office filled with green plants was a pleasant, even soothing, experience, but hardly a life-enhancing one; not so any more. Plants are a necessity these days. We depend on them to clean the air we breathe, having discovered that green plants are far more efficient at removing pollutants than any machine.

Plants absorb many harmful contaminants, such as formaldehyde, benzene, and carbon monoxide. Formaldehyde, one of the worst, is considered to be a contributing factor to the high cancer rate in the United States. Formaldehyde is found in many of the materials used in home building and furnishings, including plywood, particle board, decorative paneling, floor covering, and carpet backing. It is also found in items we regularly bring into the house, such as grocery bags, waxed bags, facial tissues, common cleaning agents, fire-retardant and permanent-press clothing, tobacco, and cooking and heating gas.

Among the most efficient air cleaners are spider plants, golden pothos, and elephant-ear philodendron. Dr. William Wolverton, formerly a senior research scientist at NASA, has calculated that fifteen to twenty of these common houseplants can clean and refresh the air in an average-sized house. Interestingly, NASA has concluded that plants become more effective at cleaning the air as pollution levels increase. It seems that in areas of low-level pollution, fewer molecules come into contact with the leaf's surface, so the benefits are not as great. Why are green plants so effective? They are natural generators of the negative ions in the air we breathe. Negative ionization promotes a feeling of well-being, of freshness, and of rejuvenation.

Negative ionization
Negative ionization increases with movement. If you walk by a waterfall, if you walk in the woods, you feel refreshed and exhilarated. The natural circulation of the water as it falls and the wind as it blows through the trees increases the amount of negative ionization in the air. When you clean a room, when you do the body rub, you are also increasing it.

An ion is a particle that can carry either a negative or a positive electrical charge. In this case, negatively charged ions are the ones we want around us. Negative ionization occurs when ions move away from the earth. It's helpful to think of negative ions as moving up and out, cleaning and refreshing everything as they go. Positive ions are those that move toward the center of the earth. Think of them as moving down and in, bringing heaviness and stagnation with them.

Any room that's not cleaned for a while will take on a dark, heavy feeling. When you open the window and pull up the shades to let in air and sunlight, when you clean the space, what you are actually doing is changing positive ions to negative ones. Fresh air, sunlight, and thorough cleaning can transform any room by infusing it with refreshed energy. Being in such a room feels wonderful. Negative ionization is big news these days. Many people are buying ionizing machines for their homes. Green plants are far cheaper and far more effective. They play a significant role in promoting good health.

Large, strong plants that grow upward are more effective than hanging plants for changing the energy in your house or office. Buy potted plants that sit on the floor. If space permits, make sure a few of them are large. A hanging plant is better than no plant at all, so, if you have a space problem, resort to using one. Use as many plants as you care to, making sure there are not so many that the room looks overcrowded or movement is hampered. You don't want your guests to feel they need a machete!

Noise Pollution

One of the unsung virtues of plants is that they protect us from noise pollution. Have you ever spent time in an evergreen forest? In 1985, I was invited to teach at a macrobiotic summer camp that was held in a pine forest north of Oslo, Norway. One day, during my free time, I went for a walk in the woods.

For some reason, it felt eerie being there. It took a while for me to realize that this was the first time I had ever experienced complete quiet. There was simply nothing to hear.

Plants have the ability to absorb sound. All plants can do this, but evergreens are especially adept at soaking up noise. If you keep a lot of plants in the house, they will help keep the noise level down. It's easier to maintain good health in a quiet house. Doors slamming, television or music blasting, and people shouting all take their toll on our health.

> "One must be out-of-doors enough to experi-
> ence wholesome reality, as ballast to thought and
> sentiment. Health requires this relaxation, this
> aimless life."
> —Henry David Thoreau

Green plants in the bedroom
The most important places in the house to keep plants are the bedroom, the kitchen, and the bathroom. Many people think plants should not be kept in the bedroom. I disagree. During the day, plants give out oxygen and take in carbon dioxide. At night, they give out carbon dioxide and take in oxygen. We need more oxygen during the day, less at night, more in summer, less in winter. This natural cycle of taking in and giving out leads to greater overall oxygen intake. Having plants in the bedroom at night helps us sleep more deeply and that means we can take in more oxygen over the course of the next day. Plants in the bedroom serve to regulate the oxygen ratio so that we receive the right amount of oxygen while we sleep. As I said earlier, the body cleans and repairs

itself during the night and our plants will be right there to aid in the nocturnal rejuvenation.

It's essential to have green plants in the kitchen. Ideally, the kitchen should be sealed off from the rest of the house so that cooking fumes and odors can be vented outside. Gas fumes generate a lot of pollution that spreads easily throughout the house. Green plants will help minimize their effect on our health. Water is one of the main sources of pollution in today's houses, so it's best to keep green plants in the bathroom as well.

Because green plants work so diligently night and day to clean the air we breathe, they deserve proper care. Actually, houseplants require only minimal attention, but they do have certain needs. They require the right amount of water at regular intervals, and they must have the appropriate light. If you place a plant in direct sunlight, make sure it's meant to have a strong exposure. Different species have different needs, so be sure to get some advice from the florist or consult a book. Keep your plants in clay pots so that their roots can breathe. Check every couple of seasons to see whether they require larger pots.

Highlights:
- The most important places for green plants are the bedroom, kitchen, bathroom, and any other room in which you spend time.
- Green plants generate negative ionization that creates a calmer, more peaceful and refreshing environment.
- Green plants enable us to be clearer, brighter, and more active during the day. Their presence promotes quiet, restful, deep sleep at night.

- Green plants are the most efficient air filtration system known, especially spider plants, golden pothos, and elephant ear philodendron.
- Choose strong, upward-growing plants over hanging ones.
- Choose plants that are hardy and easy to care for.

WEAR PURE COTTON CLOTHING NEXT TO YOUR SKIN.

The body runs on electrical impulses. Nutrition, digestion, immunity, and our nervous system all depend on electrical impulses to do their work. Because pure cotton carries less of a static electrical charge than other material, when worn directly against the skin it helps neutralize imbalances within the body. If you have an imbalance in your nervous, immune, or digestive system or in your meridians, pure cotton will help counteract that imbalance. Wearing pure cotton next to your skin is one of the quickest and easiest ways to improve and maintain your health.

Synthetics carry the strongest static electrical charge. Think of the fireworks display that occurs when you make a bed using synthetic sheets or blankets. Try making the bed with the lights off! The strong static electrical charge in synthetics interferes with the body's functioning. Synthetic fabrics make imbalances worse. Some materials that are natural to begin with go through chemical processing that produces the same effect on the body as synthetics. Rayon is a good example.

Cotton is the most neutral fabric, followed by linen, silk, and wool. Silk is natural, but its animal quality gives it a strong static charge. Wool is also natural, but it carries a much stronger charge than cotton or even silk. It's best not to wear wool directly against the skin.

Everyone, but especially people living in modern houses or high-rise apartment buildings, has an electromagnetic imbalance in his or her environment. Natural materials help lessen all imbalances. Synthetics increase, amplify, and enhance imbalances. Whatever the condition of your body or your environment, it will worsen if you wear synthetics directly against your skin. If you are feeling tired, wearing a synthetic next to your skin will increase your fatigue. If you are feeling anxious, it will make you feel more anxious. Your health problems will worsen quickly if you wear synthetics against your skin.

It is especially important to wear pure cotton underwear, bras, socks, and pajamas and to use pure cotton sheets, pillowcases, towels, and washcloths. Organic cotton is even better. If you follow this simple suggestion, you will feel more refreshed and enjoy better resistance to illness. Start by replacing your underwear and socks. It's often difficult to find all-cotton goods. Shop carefully and make sure to read the content labels. These days, even items advertised as cotton often contain a small percentage of synthetic. When you do find what suits you, keep a record of where the item was purchased. This is helpful when it's time to reorder.

Highlights:
- Cotton is a buffer that helps neutralize imbalances in the body and environment.
- Woolens and synthetics can amplify imbalances in your body and environment.

- Underwear, socks, bras, sheets, pillowcases, and towels should be 100% cotton.
- Wear cotton against the skin under clothing made from other materials.
- Try to find organic cotton.

USE NATURAL MATERIALS, WOOD, COTTON, WOOL, ETC. IN YOUR HOME.

Think of your home as a recharging station. We leave home to go to work, to shop, to go to school, or to play. We return to refresh, re-nourish, and re-balance so we have the energy and the will to leave again. If our homes and furnishings are made from natural materials, we can recharge more effectively.

It's best to have furniture made of real wood, to choose cotton for your upholstery, drapes, and curtains and wool for your carpeting. Wool carpeting is far better for your health than synthetic which, like imitation wood and plywood, is processed with formaldehyde. If you can replace the man-made materials in your home with natural ones, you will feel much more comfortable in your day-to-day life.

Natural Bedding

Try to buy 100 % organic cotton sheets. They can be expensive, so keep your eye out for sales. Avoid sheets that do not require ironing. They have been treated with formaldehyde. It's far better for your health to sleep on high-quality, wrinkled but non-toxic sheets than on smooth toxic ones. It's all a matter of priorities. Reasonably priced, high-quality, pure cotton towels and washcloths are relatively easy to find. Still, it's necessary to read the content labels carefully.

A futon is a good possible choice for a mattress. Futons are generally made of cotton and their frames of wood. Make sure the futon you buy is all-cotton. If you are not ready to change your entire bed, you can buy just the futon mattress and place it over your existing mattress or box spring. Organic latex mattresses are also a good choice. You can also buy an organic latex topper to place over your existing mattress. Conventional mattresses are made with synthetic materials (and metal as well, in the case of inner-spring mattresses), so the sooner you can replace yours with a futon, the faster your health will improve.

You will enjoy the experience of having natural materials close to you. In the beginning, it may take some effort to replace all your synthetic belongings; but after the initial outlay of energy and money, it will be easy to replace items as they wear out. Surrounding yourself with cotton is a good health habit that will help you feel and look your best.

Transparent Building

Years ago when teaching at a seminar in Switzerland, I had the privilege of spending time in a house built of completely natural materials. The concrete was free of iron so it gave off no electromagnetic charge, and the wood had been specially treated. When you were inside this house, you felt almost as if you were outdoors. It was the most transparent building environment I have ever been in. Teaching at that seminar was effortless because I was being energized all day.

Contrast that environment with that of department stores, for instance, where you are surrounded by synthetic materials and relentless fluorescent lighting. In such an environment, I very quickly become irritable. Being in man-made surroundings exhausts your body and shatters your thinking. I always feel sorry for the salespeople who have to endure this discomfort on a daily basis. Often, nowadays, there's also loud music playing. I sometimes wonder if these stores are uncomfortable on purpose. Maybe the idea is to get you to buy quickly and leave.

It's best that whatever you bring into your home be as free of chemicals and toxins as possible. Avoid using household cleaning products with high chemical content. They create their own pollution. A wide variety of excellent chemical-free cleaning products are available in health-food stores, most of which are not tested on animals.

Natural-food stores also have a large selection of self-care products, including cosmetics. Use these instead of conventional products that are full of chemicals detrimental to health, chemicals that are absorbed through the pores and into the body's organs, where they create an additional burden on the immune system. Natural products are just as effective as—and in most cases superior to—those laced with chemicals. If you are unable to find what you need in your area, you can order from any number of catalogue companies that specialize in natural products.

Fooling the Compass

I often carry a compass with me to check out different environments. I have been amazed by some of my findings. In certain apartment buildings, my compass was a full ninety degrees off! The concrete used in these buildings carries such a strong electromagnetic charge that when I was facing north my compass said I was facing east. Imagine how this distortion affects our health. If a compass can be thrown so severely out of balance, then we certainly can be too. The heart of our blood is hemoglobin, an iron-containing protein. Iron is magnetic, so our blood is profoundly affected by electromagnetic fields of energy.

Many studies have shown that electromagnetic fields are detrimental to health. Older homes, generally built with more natural materials, tend to have weaker electromagnetic fields than new ones.

At one time, I lived in a hundred-year-old Victorian farmhouse that had a very comfortable feeling. It was simply decorated, with old furniture that we liked and had gotten used to. The quality of the house and the decorations helped create a feeling of comfort and well-being. When friends visited, they often remarked on this. My point is that if we surround ourselves with natural materials, we can create a harmonious and balanced environment in which we can refresh and recharge ourselves.

How many times have you found yourself in physical surroundings that make you feel uneasy, even fidgety, without being able to understand why? It could be that you are sensitive enough to be adversely affected by unnatural surroundings. The excessive use of synthetics and chemically toxic materials is what creates this discomfort. Natural materials can help. Natural materials, such as wood, cotton, and wool, act as a buffer, helping to lessen and balance electromagnetic interference.

Things we can control

Certain things are within our control. It's best not to use microwave ovens. Their so-called acceptable levels of radiation pollute our homes. Electric blankets are very harmful.

We want to rest and recharge naturally, without interference. Electric stoves are another major source of electromagnetic radiation. I recommend that you cook with gas. If natural gas isn't available where you live, switch from electricity to propane gas. It's easy to do and convenient to use. Cooking with electricity affects the taste and consistency of food. The flavors don't harmonize naturally, and it's difficult to achieve the desired crispness. Professional chefs always choose to cook with gas.

If you have any fluorescent light bulbs in your house, replace them with incandescent or full-spectrum ones. You and your house will look much better in the glow of incandescent lighting. And your state of mind will improve. Fluorescent lighting has been proven to cause depression.

Television sets also emit harmful rays, so try to avoid spending hours sitting in front of yours. Remember that the farther away you sit from the television set, the less exposure you will receive. It's best to turn the TV off when you're not watching it, as electromagnetic fields pass through walls. Lastly, please don't put a television set in your bedroom.

I am aware that the beginning of anything can be overwhelming, and the practice of macrobiotics is no exception. Let's say that you have begun to eat good food in an orderly way, and have started your walking program and are doing the body rub and reaping its benefits. The next step is to surround yourself with materials that will enhance your sense of well-being and contribute to your overall good health.

Highlights:
- Choose natural materials when replacing home furnishings.

- Use natural wood, cotton, and wool instead of synthetic materials in your home.
- Try a futon, a natural, all-cotton mattress, for sleeping.
- Use natural cleaning products, soaps, and cosmetics.
- Stop using microwave ovens and electric blankets.
- Cook with natural, propane, or even butane gas. Please do not cook with electricity.
- Watch television sparingly.

MAKE YOUR MACROBIOTIC PRACTICE WORK

KEEPING TO THE FORMAT OF MEALS IMPROVES YOUR ABILITY TO MAKE HEALTHFUL FOOD CHOICES. GOOD EATING HABITS, STEPS ONE AND TWO, ARE THE CONTROLLING FACTORS IN GOOD HEALTH.

The biggest mistake
The sixth step incorporates the essence of each of the five previous steps. The point here is that by keeping to the Format of Meals, we automatically have clear guidelines as to wise food choices under any and all circumstances, whether we're eating at home, in a restaurant, or on an airplane. As I said earlier, the biggest mistake most people make is to focus on Diet: Content and Quality rather than on Eating Habits: Format of Meals. Eating Habits are what keep us on track.

Eating home versus eating out

Food choices that are clear when we eat at home can seem murky when we eat out. When we're at home, we can choose the highest-quality organically grown short-grain brown rice, organic vegetables, the best-quality miso and so on. If we are at the mercy of a mediocre restaurant, we might order white rice and steamed broccoli (possibly even frozen). The quality is lower, yes, but the Format is intact. We have a grain and a vegetable on our plate. Quality can always be adjusted up or down depending on where we find ourselves. Of course, the degree of the adjustment depends on our condition. We must ask: "What can my health afford at this time? How liberal can I be?"

As simple as this might sound, most people see little or no connection between meals at home and meals outside the home. At home they take care to make good choices but when they eat out they often throw away the guidelines, meaning the Format of Meals, and choose whatever appeals to them. This is a serious mistake. The Format is what helps us maintain our direction toward health. If, however, we believe Content and Quality are more important than Format and we can't get organic short-grain rice, the temptation is to abandon the Format as well. Once we create a separation in our minds between what we eat at home and what we eat outside, it follows that we begin to see food in terms of black and white. We think, "I ate something I shouldn't have, I'm off the diet, I'm in trouble, I can never eat out, this is too hard." But, really, if we focus on the Format wherever we are, we will automatically make the wisest choices possible and we will continue to move in the direction of health.

The second biggest mistake

Let's look at maintaining the direction toward health from another angle: structure (another word for Format) versus variety. The second biggest mistake most people make is to allow the structure, which should be tight, to become loose. Once that happens, the need for variety diminishes and eventually changes to a pattern of repetition, a pattern that directs us away from health. If the legs of a table are loose, the table can be said to have a wobbly structure. It can barely support itself. If we remove the legs altogether, the table will collapse completely. Or to use Nature's model once again, the sun rises and sets every day, a phenomenon that is part of the structure of the universe. If the sun doesn't rise or set, it's all over for the planet. In the same way, once we let the structure or Format go, we set ourselves on a path away from health.

Here are the main danger signals:
- You don't sit down and take time for your meals.
- You do other things while eating.
- Your mealtimes become irregular.
- You stop having a grain and vegetable with every meal.

How does this work? Let's say you want to have lunch at twelve-thirty, no later than one o'clock, but you're too busy to eat. By the time you do eat, your appetite is completely altered because your blood sugar has fallen. Low blood sugar means that in order to feel satisfied, either you have to eat more than usual—in other words, overeat—or you have to have something sweet. It follows that, once having eaten a late lunch, you have no appetite for dinner at the regular time. If you keep to your regular dinnertime but eat less than usual, an hour or two later you'll want a snack. Or, instead of dinner at six, let's say you decide to eat at eight-thirty. Either way, you won't have three full hours between dinner and bedtime since you have to go to bed at a reasonable hour in order to get up early the next morning. You don't sleep very well that night (no one sleeps well on a full stomach). It's difficult to get up the next morning and, when you do drag yourself out of bed, you don't feel refreshed. You can see how one change in the structure or Format inevitably leads to another and how, in the end, these changes will lead you away from health.

Although having a grain and vegetable with every meal comes under the heading of Diet, there is an overlap with Format. The meal you sit down to eat must qualify as a meal, meaning it must contain a grain or grain product and a vegetable. When you stop having both a grain and a vegetable with every meal, most commonly that meal is breakfast and it's the vegetable that disappears from the plate. If you've reached this stage, you can pretty much assume you've begun to lose your direction. You're getting way off track.

Balance and imbalance perpetuate themselves

One of the guiding principles of life is that balance perpetuates itself. And, as you might suspect, imbalance perpetuates itself as well. As you let go of more and more of the structure, you start to feel more and more pressure. You might believe the buildup of pressure comes from having to market, prepare, and cook the food or from the pressure of having to eat at a regular time—but I don't think so. I think the reverse is true. The usual pattern is that you feel rushed, so you begin to rush your meals. The more we rush our meals, the more rushed we feel. Sitting down and taking time for meals actually eases pressure. If you think of a meal as a time for recharging, reorienting, and regaining balance, if no matter how stressed you feel you take the time to sit down, eat slowly, and chew well, when you finish eating you will feel refreshed and calm. Any decisions you make in this frame of mind are bound to be wiser than those made under pressure.

Some people find it helpful to think of chewing as a form of meditation, somewhat like breathing practices. The result in both cases is heightened mental and emotional clarity and a feeling of deep calm. Remember, it's important to come to the table prepared to chew. Before you sit down, ask yourself "What are my priorities?" If good health is one of them, then take time for your meal, eat your food slowly, and chew it well.

Structure Versus Variety

Let's go back to structure versus variety. I said earlier that when the structure becomes loose, the need for variety diminishes—or we could say, tightens—and eventually repetition replaces variety altogether. In effect, polarity is reversed. What do I mean by this? Let me start with a basic premise: the more we seek variety, the more nutrition we get from our food. If we eat the same few foods over and over again, eventually not much happens. If someone repeats the same thing over and over again, eventually you stop hearing what is being said. It goes in one ear and out the other. It's no different with food. In one end and out the other—without much benefit.

Unfortunately, often we don't notice that this is happening. It's difficult to be aware of what we're eating day to day. Food is the closest thing to us, so we don't have the advantage of perspective. We think we have variety—we eat blanched, steamed, and sautéed vegetables daily; we eat different grains, oatmeal, brown rice, millet, barley—where's the repetition in all this? Every morning we have oatmeal and steamed kale; for lunch we have rice and blanched broccoli and cabbage; for dinner miso soup, rice with sesame seeds, sautéed mixed vegetables, pressed salad with napa cabbage. Isn't that variety? No. It's repetition. Taking several dishes and repeating them day after day after day is repetition. Having blanched broccoli and cabbage every day for lunch is repetition. Having oatmeal for breakfast every morning is repetition.

Appetite is stimulated by variety. Variety also creates satisfaction. If we lack variety in both ingredients and preparation, we don't feel satisfied with our food, and so we overeat at mealtimes and snack before bed.

Highlights:
- Good eating habits, steps one and two, are the controlling factors in good health.
- Good eating habits increase your ability to make healthy choices.
- When traveling or eating out, keep to the format of grains and vegetables as the basis of a meal. Quality can be adjusted up or down. White rice or commercial pasta is a better choice than going without a grain.
- Commercial vegetable soup is a better choice than no soup at all.

KEEP A DAILY MENU BOOK TO HELP YOU BECOME MORE OBJECTIVE ABOUT YOUR MACROBIOTIC PRACTICE.

Underlying everything in this book so far is the basic question, how do we keep moving in the direction of health? Keeping a menu book—or a journal, if you prefer to call it that—is the best way I know of. It's very difficult to be aware of what we're doing day to day, especially with regard to diet. As I've said before, food is the closest thing to us, so it's hard to be objective. The power of a menu book is that it lets you see if you are really getting enough variety.

Enter the date, time, and menu for every meal, snack, or nibble that passes your lips, along with a brief comment on how you felt that day. Review your menu book every so often and reflect on its contents. It's difficult to be objective when you are entering information. Objectivity comes later. In this way, you will know whether or not you are getting variety. Keeping a daily menu book takes the guesswork out of tracking the changes in your health. (It's not necessary to include recipes, although you may if you wish.)

Your menu book can be as simple or as detailed as you care to make it. Some people keep track of their daily functions as well as their daily food—bowel movements, bedtime, sleep patterns, moods, and so on. Looking back, you can see how you were feeling physically, mentally, and emotionally on any given day. Then you can begin to correlate what you ate or did on a particular day with how you felt that day. For instance: I did this and I felt really good—my thinking was clear, I ate this and I didn't feel very well, I did this and I was irritable, I did that and I was really tired. You can't learn this sort of thing in school. How certain foods, patterns, and behaviors affect you can only be self-taught. If you write just a sentence or two every day, that should be enough to jog your memory and help you discover whether you are really doing what you think you're doing. I can't stress enough the importance of keeping a menu book. It's one way to measure how serious your commitment is to improving and strengthening your health.

I must confess that I've never really kept a menu book; but in the past, during the years when I was teaching several times a week, I kept a kind of journal. I entered the outline of every lecture I gave along with some comments, no matter how often I lectured on the same topic. It's interesting to look back over these journals. There are times when I thought my condition was good and my thinking orderly, but my journal shows otherwise. Or, looking back at other periods when my notes indicate that my condition was off, I can see by the outline of my lecture that my thinking was very clear and orderly. The point is that when you're in the throes of doing something, it's nearly impossible to be objective. But when you look back, you can often see the truth.

One final comment on this point: You might think you don't need to do this, you're an experienced cook, you don't need to improve your cooking. Let me assure you that even experienced, longtime macrobiotic cooks keep menu books. I can guarantee that if you keep one, your practice will improve, as will your cooking. Objectivity is the key. You can see where you've fallen short or gone overboard.

Highlights:
- Keep a hard or spiral-bound book in your kitchen to record your menus and snacks.

- Keep notes on your activities, symptoms, and general feelings.
- Refer back to previous days, weeks, and months to see any patterns that emerge from your practice.
- Keeping a daily menu book is one of the best ways to improve your practice and discover your mistakes.
- Such a journal allows you to evaluate your practice and its benefits more objectively.

STEP 7

CULTIVATE THE SPIRIT OF HEALTH

The seventh step is the one that completes the other six, the one without which the other six remain mechanical and, in a sense, external to us, animated by willpower rather than love. What is too often missing from current macrobiotic practice is the spirit of health itself. It's taken me a long time to work out how to convey the essence of this spirit—one that is inseparable from the theory and practice of macrobiotics. Lacking this spirit, we can never make the transition to lasting health.

Please bear with me as I repeat once again: health is a direction, a condition we move toward day by day throughout life. Sickness is also a direction. Depending on the totality of our eating habits, diet, and daily lifestyle practices, we move in one direction or the other. It should be no surprise then that if we follow the macrobiotic guidelines accurately, we move toward health. If we ignore them, we move toward sickness. Let me state something unequivocally: health is a condition we grow into throughout our lives. This is a very important point. Today, the most commonly held belief is that we start out in life with a certain amount of health—call it our capital—that we spend as we age until, in a manner of speaking, we are bankrupt. Now, to believe that aging is a fate that brings, among other things, the loss of bones, teeth, beautiful skin, flexibility, memory, and the ability to enjoy and fully participate in life—that this fate is as sure as death and taxes—is a very heavy burden to bear. Yet this belief is so strong that everyone who can afford to carries the financial burden of a lifetime of health insurance.

Is this kind of deterioration really the human fate? I don't think so. Is the aging process I have just described based on a natural model of aging—of living in harmony with Nature— or is it simply the experience of those who live an anti-natural lifestyle? I think you know the answer. Let me assure you that it is not natural to deteriorate with age. If you look at Nature's model—take for instance, trees—what do you see? Once the aptly named "mighty oak" has grown to fullness, then seedlings sprout and when these seedlings need more light and more space to continue growing, the oak passes on. In other words, when the oak has fulfilled its destiny, it moves on.

> "A wise man should consider that health is the greatest of human blessings, and learn how by his own thought to derive the benefit from his illness."
> —Hippocrates

In the past, people readily moved on when they had had enough of life. It was that simple. (In fact, the novels of the nineteenth century are filled with death-bed scenes involving characters who, having reached this point, put their affairs in order, paid their debts, said their farewells to family and friends, and either sat down or lay down and died.) They chose the time and place of their death. They died not of sickness but because they had had enough of life. Some of you might have had parents or grandparents who were able to do this. Odd though it might seem to us, it's really no different from anything else we've had enough of in life. No matter how much we enjoy something, eventually we reach a point of satiation where more isn't going to add to the experience. In fact, it may well detract from it. We can have the best conversation, the best meal, the best vacation, whatever. Still, sooner or later, we get to the point of fullness and satisfaction. We've had enough. It's time to move on. It's a sign of spiritual maturity to know when that time is.

For the first eighteen to twenty years after birth, we grow our bodies. At that point, the body should stop growing—in terms of weight as well as height. Our natural weight is achieved somewhere between the ages of sixteen and twenty. People new to macrobiotics are sometimes quite heavy. The prospect of losing weight appeals to them, but often they lose more than they are comfortable with. I always ask, "How much did you weigh when you were sixteen? How much did you weigh when you got your first driver's license? That's your natural weight, and that's probably what you'll end up weighing." They become alarmed. "That's too thin," they say. No, it's not too thin. Let me explain. As I said, we spend the first part of life growing the body. At birth, the body is not completely formed. The nervous system is not fully developed, nor are the lungs, immune system, or bones. We take the next sixteen to twenty years to grow these, after which we stop growing physically and begin to grow mentally and spiritually. That is, we begin to grow our consciousness.

> "Dwell not upon thy weariness, thy strength shall be according to the measure of thy desire."
> —Arabian Proverb

Health itself has three aspects: physical, mental, and spiritual. Physical health is the foundation of mental and spiritual health. When we have good vitality, good energy, then we sleep well. If we sleep well, then we are alert and our memory is excellent. We don't anger easily. We are filled with a deep sense of joy and appreciation. On the other hand, with limited physical vitality, sleep isn't usually sound or refreshing, memory is unreliable, and there is a tendency to become easily irritated. Worst of all, joy and alertness are lost, along with feelings of gratitude for life itself.

As I said, the first part of life is devoted to the growth of the body and the creation of a high degree of physical health. Physical health is the foundation for the growth and nourishment of mental and spiritual health. When you look at traditional societies, you see that they valued their elders for their life's experience and their ability to guide younger people. Think about it, if the elders were incapable of guiding their own lives because of impaired memory and physical debilitation, how could they guide anyone else? Why would anyone seek them out? The answer is that the memory of the elders *didn't* deteriorate. On the contrary, it increased with age. Their patience with life itself, their joy, their appreciation for all of life, their understanding of the relationship between difficulty and happiness—all these increased and flowered as they aged. Just as the flower represents the culmination of the growth process of a plant, the final maturation before passing on to the next stage, in the same way old age should be the flowering of our life on earth.

What we refer to when we talk about health these days—health being merely an absence of serious illness—is a very recent model. The world's health began to deteriorate at the time of the Industrial Revolution, but the definitive turning point was World War II.

It's most important that we reexamine our definition of health itself. We must ask ourselves what health is and what we need to do to develop it so that old age is once again a flowering. One thing that does change with age is that we become less interested in sensory experience and more interested in social matters. We become more interested in discovering for ourselves the meaning of life—that is, in discovering what we came here to do so that we can complete the task, so that one day we can honestly say we are satisfied, we have had enough of this life.

> "And man dies and is buried, and all his words
> and actions are forgotten, but the food he has
> eaten lives after him in the sound or rotten bones
> of his children."
>
> —George Orwell

I'd have to say, based on my years of counseling so many seriously ill older people, that most of them never did what they really wanted to with their lives. They were waiting until retirement to make their dreams a reality, but once retired they found they didn't want to do anything. Almost inevitably what followed was a very rapid physical and mental deterioration. It's almost axiomatic that doing what we really want to do day to day is what nourishes life and health. Those activities that we never grow tired of, that we don't want to retire from, that, in effect, never end for us, are life and health giving. Work we love is a form of play. If we live this way, then, like the elders of traditional eras, when we are ready to hand the baton off to someone else we will do it with gratitude and in the spirit of adventure.

Let's start here: we are all guided by our consciousness. If our consciousness keeps telling us that we are going to get sick and die, then that's generally what happens. But if our consciousness is constantly guiding us toward health, health is what we get. A genuinely healthy person has more energy, more vitality, and a greater interest in life as he or she ages. I have seen it over and over. We all have this capacity.

I have spent the greater part of my adult life trying to create the guidelines that will help those who are interested achieve the kind of health I have been describing. Let's examine the seventh step or last guideline in more detail.

"Dream lofty dreams, and as you dream, so shall you become."

– James Allen

BE OPEN AND CURIOUS AND CULTIVATE AN ENDLESS APPRECIATION FOR ALL OF LIFE.

Everyone likes to look at healthy children. Why do you suppose that is? For one thing, their faces are open and clear, not closed and clouded with conceptual thinking, bad experiences, and heavy responsibilities. Since they don't have to get up in the morning and work at jobs they hate, their faces reflect an incredible openness and sense of curiosity. This openness is the source of their energy. When you look at a child, you see bright freshness. The same sort of freshness you see when you look at a healthy plant. A healthy plant is one that is getting the proper nourishment. The soil, water, sunlight, breeze, temperature—everything is suitable. We can say the plant has good nourishment and good circulation. When we look at a healthy child, we see the same thing. Healthy children can eat very, very little or they can eat a lot, or they can eat very simple food and still grow very well. The reason for this is that they have good digestion, meaning they are able to absorb nutrition very efficiently from whatever amount of food they eat. At the same time, they have excellent circulation. They can go out in the coldest weather with almost no clothing on and they don't feel the cold. Their circulation is so good that they have no hardness in their bodies. You can bend children, twist them like pretzels, and the more you do this the funnier they think it is.

"Gratitude is the heart's memory."
—French Proverb

We can see this very clearly by looking at plants. If their nourishment, temperature, or circulation is off, plants react very quickly by losing their freshness. If you over-water, they become limp and lifeless; if you under-water, they become hard, dry, and inflexible. What I am trying to convey with this analogy is that openness or freshness, curiosity, and appreciation mean that we are connected to Nature, connected to life itself—or to God, if you prefer to say it that way. The benefits of a good connection are good nourishment and good circulation.

Experts today are concerned about children's lack of activity. As I mentioned earlier, we are in the midst of a nationwide epidemic of juvenile obesity as well as juvenile diabetes. Parents are being urged to take their children outside and play with them. Isn't this a strange idea? When I was a kid, our parents couldn't get us to come indoors, even for meals. It was a constant battle. There is something really wrong when kids don't want to play. Before children were told that they had to exercise to be healthy, they had the best exercise in the world—play—but once they were introduced to it as a concept, they no longer wanted to exercise at all. Today, children's minds are infected with unhealthy ideas from many sources. Their minds are full of junk ideas, their bodies full of junk food. The inevitable result is a loss of openness and circulation. All of a sudden, it's too cold or too hot to go outside. Minds and bodies close and become inflexible and our children no longer have the openness, freshness, and curiosity they had just two or three years earlier.

> "Plant a kernel of wheat and you reap a pint; plant a pint and you reap a bushel. Always the law works to give you back more than you give."
> —Anthony Norvell

The way for anyone to recover openness and curiosity is to consciously practice gratitude and appreciation. This practice opens the mind and the heart. When we complain, blame, and criticize, we close our minds. You can say we close ourselves off to life itself or to Nature or to God. Let me give you an example of what I mean. In the early years of my practice, I had a client with colon cancer who had refused surgery. This man, who was a concentration camp survivor, had an iron will. For a year and a half, he ate everything I recommended. After the first nine months, he went to have a checkup with the doctor who had diagnosed him. When the doctor couldn't find any trace of the cancer, he assumed he had misdiagnosed the case. My client continued to practice macrobiotics for another nine months. Then one day I got a phone call from his son. He told me his father had begun to eat other sorts of food and was having health problems again. I suggested that his father return to my original recommendations. The son called back and told me his father was refusing to eat the macrobiotic way, that he would rather die than continue to eat the food. And that's what happened. He ate the macrobiotic way for eighteen months, but during all that time he failed to develop a sense of gratitude or appreciation for what had been given to him. I know it sounds harsh, but I have seen this kind of response again and again in my thirty-odd years of counseling. The man with colon cancer was so strong-willed that he would have eaten sawdust for a year and a half if I had recommended it. Yet because he didn't develop a deep sense of appreciation, the food that gave him back his life never became delicious to him.

> "To speak gratitude is courteous and pleasant, to enact gratitude is generous and noble, but to live gratitude is to touch heaven."
> —Johannes A. Gaertner

Let's say there's a man you like, someone you appreciate, and that person does something you're not too crazy about. You don't drop him. Since you're fond of him and appreciate his qualities, you don't give too much weight to what he's done. You cut him some slack. However, if you aren't open to him to start with and, as a consequence, can't appreciate his finer qualities, then what he's just done becomes a huge impediment and chances are you'll drop him altogether.

What I'm getting at is this: Appreciation shows openness. If we're open to someone, we see more and more of their good qualities. If we're closed, we see more and more of their negative ones. Appreciation is an expression of our openness to life, our willingness to receive life itself. And that openness manifests itself day to day in a deep interest in and curiosity about life, about everything—food, friendship, love, sex, adventures, travel, history, and so on.

"Take only memories, leave nothing but footprints."
—Chief Seattle

BE FLEXIBLE AND ADAPTABLE IN YOUR PRACTICE.
There are only two ways I know of that will help you keep your practice flexible and adaptable. One is to establish a deep connection with the source of life and renewal that is the natural world. You can do this by practicing the seven steps really well. The other is to keep in touch with new developments in macrobiotic thinking. Everything changes over time. Everything adapts or dies. Nothing is fixed in cement, including macrobiotics. In today's rapidly changing world, adaptability and flexibility are more important than ever before. Those people who have been practicing for five, ten, twenty years

and haven't adapted their ways of cooking and eating to the changing conditions of life inevitably get into trouble. We have to look carefully at what we're doing on a daily basis. If we can't recognize an imbalance in ourselves—and it's very hard to see in oneself—then we should seek guidance.

Of course, the degree of flexibility you can permit yourself depends on your health and the circumstances in which you find yourself. Health is freedom. The better your health, the more relaxed you can afford to be socially. If your health can't afford it, then no matter what the situation or circumstance is, it's better not to mess around. If you're healthy, one binge won't harm you; but if you have a serious health problem and you've been practicing well, one binge can cause devastation. If health were money and you were making five hundred dollars a week, then a thousand-dollar car repair would represent serious damage to your financial health. But if you were making ten thousand a week, it would be no big deal.

Ideally, of course, it would be wonderful if everyone could eat very carefully day to day and be adaptable and flexible socially when appropriate. To be able to do this depends on your degree of health. My hope is that you make yourself healthy as quickly as possible so you can do what you want. Let me repeat that health is freedom. People think that freedom produces more freedom, but I don't agree. I prefer to use words like order or structure rather than discipline, but the meaning is the same. Freedom rests on and comes out of discipline.

"When you're finished changing, you're finished."
—Benjamin Franklin

Where is it most important to exercise discipline, in our Eating Habits or in our Diet? Do we exercise discipline by making sure we sit down to eat, take time for meals, have a grain and vegetable with every meal, etc., or do we exercise it by thinking, I can eat this, I can't eat that? The answer, of course, is we apply discipline with respect to our Eating Habits. For most people, diet is not discipline. If we enjoy the food, we look forward to eating it. In my book, that's not discipline.

One last point: please try to be flexible and adaptable not only in your own practice but also in your dealings with your children, partners, relatives, and friends.

DEVELOP A STRONG WILL AND THE DETERMINATION TO CREATE YOUR OWN HEALTH.

The will to create enduring health has to come from within. No matter how loving, generous, and helpful family and friends are, this is a gift they cannot give us. My long-time observation is that people who want to become well do just that. I am always being asked, "Can macrobiotics help cure my illness?" But the question should be, "Can macrobiotics help me cure myself?" It's the person who determines the outcome, not the disease, just as it's the person who determines what illness he or she will get. Have you ever wondered why it is that we get one sort of illness and not another? Based on my counseling experience, I can tell you that we get only that type of illness or disease that perfectly fits our nature. Why should this be the case? Think about it. Becoming ill is an indication—an alarm-bell, in some cases—that we've gotten way off-track, that we are seriously out of balance. And we each get out of balance in our own particular way. The type of illness we contract tells us what we need to learn about ourselves in order to get back on track.

"Valor consists in the power of self-recovery."
—Ralph Waldo Emerson

If we are open and appreciative, then we can understand the significance of the illness in our lives, and we can change. If not, then we will just go on repeating the behavior that brought us the illness in the first place. Those who have overcome a terminal illness all say the same thing. "My illness was the best thing that ever happened to me. It changed my life."

"It is idle to say that men are not responsible for their misfortunes."
—Samuel Butler

Some years ago, I invited a young couple from Philadelphia to be part of a panel discussion I led after a lecture I gave at a natural-foods convention. The husband had had testicular cancer many years before and had refused to have his testicle removed surgically. In the beginning, he didn't practice macrobiotics consistently well. He'd visit me, practice well for a while, and then ease up. Well, the cancer spread, it put pressure on his kidneys, and he nearly died. He had to have serious, heavy-duty chemotherapy. He recovered, but his doctors claimed that the spread was due to my interference in his medical treatment. He said, "No, he gave me good advice but I didn't take it. This was entirely my fault." At any rate, his doctors told him he would be sterile. It's important to know that throughout this long ordeal, he never gave up practicing his version of macrobiotics. I assured him that if he could bring himself to practice really well, he could overcome the sterility. I'm happy to tell you the couple has three strong, healthy children. During the panel discussion, his wife said, "My husband's cancer was the best thing that ever happened to us. Without it, we wouldn't have found the macrobiotic way of life and we wouldn't have had such wonderful children," one of whom is a highly gifted pianist. I was used to hearing such remarks from the person who'd been ill, but this was the first time I had ever heard—and from a spouse—that macrobiotics was the best thing that had ever happened to an entire family.

"Who is strong? He that can conquer his bad habits."
—Benjamin Franklin

BE ACCURATE IN YOUR PRACTICE.

Accuracy is a spiritual practice, plain and simple. If we are accurate in our practice, it means that we have the ability to devote ourselves to something, to be with something completely without any separation, without any distraction. It means that we understand the value of small things and how the small relates to the large, how the part relates to the whole. So often, it's the little things in life that make a difference. It's been said, and rightly so, that God is in the details. For example, we can make the most wonderful dish in the world, but if we don't season it properly, it won't come to life, it won't taste delicious even though everything up to the point of seasoning was done well. The point at which we add salt to a dish determines the degree of flavor the dish will have, whether it will taste salty or sweet. In this case, accurate timing is crucial.

To practice the macrobiotic way of life accurately means you must pay attention. You must give your undivided attention to sitting down to eat, to chewing well, to getting variety, to doing the body rub, and so on. To pay attention means to be there, mind, body, and spirit—with no separation—in the moment you are doing these things. Accuracy is something that is learned by example and training very early in life. If we haven't had the good fortune to learn it then, we have to work hard to recover our ability to be accurate. And this ability is often the deciding factor in whether or not we recover. Accuracy is a condition of body, mind, and spirit. It is a spiritual practice, not a mechanical one.

"When walking, walk. When eating, eat."
—Zen Proverb

My father was a diamond setter. He taught only two people, my cousin and myself, although there were many others who wanted to learn the trade at that time. When you apprenticed yourself to him, your first job was to sweep the floors, sweep them well and sweep them endlessly, because the bits of precious metals and gems that had fallen to the floor in the course of the work had to be recovered. Almost everybody failed the sweeping test. They couldn't or didn't want to learn to sweep accurately. If they couldn't be accurate when sweeping, my father wouldn't teach them anything more. He'd say, "They're not worth teaching. They can't even sweep the floor." His thinking was, if you're going to do something, do it well or don't do it at all.

Accuracy regarding the seemingly smallest and most meaningless tasks—that is, the willingness, the patience and the ability to do the most meaningless thing fully and completely—is a quality that fewer and fewer people seem to value. Yet those living in spiritual communities, such as monasteries, willingly undertake the most menial chores and do them with appreciation and joy, understanding that it is through this work that they will grow spiritually. If you find it difficult to be accurate, then perhaps one way to develop this quality would be to take on more and more menial tasks and do them with a full heart. Try it and see. The more accurate and precise you can be in your practice, the more you will receive from your efforts—across the board.

Now, although I use the word "accurate," often the client will substitute the word "strict." I want to be clear about this— accuracy and strictness are two entirely different qualities. For one person, to eat simply is accurate. For another, to eat widely is accurate. For some, to eat in restaurants is accurate. For others, to stay away from restaurants is accurate. Accuracy and strictness are not connected in any way; but often when people hear "accuracy," they interpret it as strictness. Strictness is a straight path to rigidity and rigidity, is a condition of hardness.

> "Good timber does not grow with ease. The
> stronger the wind, the stronger the trees."
> —J. Willard Marriot

Please, think about the meaning of the word accuracy and about how to be accurate. Accuracy implies flexibility and adaptability according to the circumstances. It's impossible to be accurate if you don't know what the requirements are. Part of learning to be accurate is to find out what the requirements are. They might involve attending classes, reading books, and so on—in other words, taking the time to find out whatever it is you really need to do to develop that quality of mind, body, and spirit we call accuracy.

CREATE A GOOD SUPPORT NETWORK.

The need to create a good support network is greater than ever. So much of what we have to learn can only be transmitted personally. In the old days, serious students had the attractive option of living in study houses. Most of us who are still actively teaching macrobiotics spent time living in study houses—six months, a year, five years—where we lived and breathed the subject. We roomed together, studied together, played together, cooked for each other, and ate together. The focus of life in the study house was to deepen one's understanding of all aspects of the macrobiotic way. The sort of education we got was very different from what most people have access to today.

Short of a study house, what can you do to create a support network? All of us need to find ways to be around healthy macrobiotic people. If among your friends or acquaintances there's a macrobiotic family that knows how to practice well, try to spend time with them. If you live in a major city, chances are you can find a macrobiotic community there. Information of this sort is sometimes posted on health-food-store bulletin boards. If you live in a more remote area, the best thing you can do is to attend major macrobiotic programs at least a few times a year—even if you have to travel great distances to get to them. Doing this will make all the difference in your practice and your health. Being in a group of people who are healthy really picks you up. There's a group dynamic that works to everyone's benefit. Your health will improve more rapidly than it would on your own, no matter how well you are practicing. And if your practice has deteriorated because of isolation, you will be inspired to clean up your act.

When I first established my school, The Strengthening Health Institute, the program consisted of two non-residential weekends. I soon realized that for the program to become more effective, it had to be residential. Students need to feel they are part of the school; they need to be involved at every level. I wanted to recreate the experience I had had of living and breathing macrobiotics, and that's very difficult to achieve if students arrive in the morning and leave in the evening. Macrobiotic study programs generally offer a traditional learning structure. As with martial-arts schools, there is usually a mix of new and experienced students, something along the lines of a one-room schoolhouse where different grades are taught together and a bit like the structure in large families where the older children typically help the younger ones.

Please do whatever it takes to create your network. Without one, it is much harder to move in the direction of health.

LEARN TO COOK WELL.

Finally, learn to cook well. I can't emphasize this enough. Macrobiotic food has a bad reputation. Many people think the food is terrible. Well, it all depends on your experience. If your first macrobiotic meal is bad, it's easy to dismiss all macrobiotic food. It's useful to remember that the world is full of bad cooks—no matter what sort of food they are preparing. And macrobiotics is no exception. However, a bad macrobiotic meal may be worse for you than an ordinary meal! Unrefined, organic grains and vegetables carry more *ki* (energy) than their counterparts. They store more energy and vitality. If macrobiotic food is well prepared, it nourishes you more than ordinary food. The down side is that if it's poorly prepared, the effects stay with you longer. We can say that macrobiotic cuisine has the potential to be the most delicious or the most dreadful of any cuisine.

> "Good cooking does not depend on whether the dish is large or small, expensive or economical. If one has the art, then a piece of celery or salted cabbage can be made into a marvelous delicacy; whereas if one has not the art, not all the greatest delicacies and rarities of land, sea or sky are of any avail."
>
> —Yuan Mei

Please remember that no one's cooking is perfect. Perfection is not the point and it's not our goal. Even the best cooks falter. What we strive for is the ability to express ourselves accurately through our cooking, in the same way that artists express themselves accurately through their art. I don't think anyone will dispute that cooking is an art. What's more, cooking is a form of art that creates life. And what is art, if not the expression of one's personal vision of life on earth? Our ability to stay with macrobiotics—and not just to stay with it but to embrace it with a full heart, to choose it enthusiastically over all other ways of life—depends a lot on how well we learn to cook. Whether we cook every day or periodically, we should know how to cook well. The more we know about what it takes to put a delicious macrobiotic meal on the table, the more appreciative we can be of the efforts of others.

I've observed over the years that there seem to be two different takes on the subject of macrobiotic food. The basic one, and the one I subscribe to, is that the food itself is delicious. Our job is to learn how to bring out its natural taste, color, and texture, using simple ingredients and traditional techniques. Simple ingredients and proper techniques are all we need to produce a delicious, satisfying meal. In this style of cooking, modeled after Japanese temple cooking, seasoning, spices, and oil are used sparingly but to great effect.

Then there's the other approach. The thinking behind it goes something like this: "I'll put up with this food for now, but once I get healthy I'll be able to eat the good stuff. I'll be able to eat more widely." There's nothing wrong, per se, with eating widely or with eating simply. It all depends on our condition. What's wrong is the implication that once we can use more oil, once we can cook with herbs and spices, once we can eat tropical fruits and vegetables, then we'll be practicing the "real" macrobiotics and our food will be truly delicious.

This is simply not true. Furthermore, what's particularly unsettling about this approach is the belief that the simple meals we eat day to day are not the most delicious, satisfying, nourishing, or fulfilling ones we can have. I think this is a dangerous approach. There is nothing more delicious than well-prepared brown rice or miso soup or blanched, steamed, or sautéed vegetables. On what do I base my assertion? The test for me is how many days in a row, how many years in a row I can eat a particular food and continue to find it delicious, satisfying, and nourishing. Now, we've all gone to fine restaurants and thought the food was incredible and said, "That was one of the best meals I've ever had." I translate such a statement to mean that if we eat such a meal once a year, it does taste that delicious. But if we eat it once a month, it tastes a bit less delicious. And, if we eat it weekly, well—you get the picture. If we eat such a meal every day, it's a safe bet that we won't be able to stand the sight or smell of it after a while. It's just too much. It's an assault on our senses. What this means to me is that such a meal is not truly delicious. Of course, from time to time, it's wonderful to have such a meal. It's a bit like describing someone as a great person and then saying you can only take that person in limited doses—which is quite different from saying "This is a great person, someone I really want to spend lots of time with."

> "Cook it with pleasure—eat it with joy."
> —Clarissa Dickson Wright

The problem is that learning to bring out the truly delicious natural taste of food without relying on such things as herbs and spices to take up the slack takes more time, patience, sensitivity, and skill than other sorts of cooking. Here's a generalization I think is valid: since I've been involved in macrobiotics, I've observed that you can divide people practicing macrobiotics into two groups. Those who, when they come up against a problem, look inward and those who, in the same circumstances, look outward. The ones who look outward don't last. (Actually, they don't last at anything.) Let's say they become dissatisfied with one or more aspects of the macrobiotic way of life—the philosophy, the healthcare, the spirituality, the cooking, whatever—it doesn't really matter. Eventually we all meet with resistance. We come up against the brick wall of ourselves, so to speak. It's part of living. And then we have two basic choices. We can look outward and think "Someone out there has got to get me past this, someone has got to help me or I'm out of here." Or we can look inward and think "I already have the means to help myself. If I just stick with this, I'll get through it." Inevitably, we all arrive at that point of resistance in our cooking. We find ourselves thinking "Is this all there is, no more ingredients, no more choices?" I can guarantee this will happen to you. When it does, if you stop and ask yourself "What can I do to make my food more delicious and exciting?" a new dimension will open up and you will be able to take your cooking to the next level. This is how the process of growth works.

If we look outside ourselves for the answer, then we relinquish the ability and the power to create or change our lives. This doesn't mean that we have to do everything by ourselves, that we can't ask for help. At one time or another, we all need guides; but we are the ones who choose them. We are the ones who decide when we need help and for how long a time. We might decide we need shiatsu massage or that we want to improve our cooking or that we have to learn more about macrobiotic philosophy so that we can better help ourselves. This frame of mind is the polar opposite of someone who thinks "This person is going to help me" or "that person is going to save my life." That's dependence. We are moving toward freedom.

Everything I've been saying comes down to this: a healthy person is self-reliant and self-sufficient. My approach to life has always been that if we're here, we already have what we need to take care of all our problems. We might require help from time to time to get past a rough spot or to have something pointed out to us or to give us a little push. But, still, it's up to us to choose what we want to do and how much energy we want to give it. It's up to us to take the initiative in our own lives. In other words, it's up to us to behave in a self-sufficient manner, and that means not waiting around for someone or something "out there" to come to our aid. Modern life encourages dependence. Part of the macrobiotic journey or adventure—for it is an adventure—is to free ourselves of that dependence by learning to develop our own healing ability and, through struggle, to gain the power to create the life we want.

> "A good cook is like a sorceress who dispenses happiness."
>
> —Elsa Schiaparelli

For many of us today, the principal issue is one of health. The challenge is how to create good health so that we are free to live our lives. But let's not forget that health is guided by spirit. And it is in the spirit of macrobiotics to look at the challenges and difficulties that come our way as gifts. For it is in meeting challenges and in overcoming difficulties that we begin to develop the power to heal ourselves, the power to build the life we want. To be truly healthy, we have to embrace the spirit of health.

Which brings me to my final point. Although the spirit of health has many components, it would be a grave mistake to forget the totality. We cannot separate one part from any of the others without destroying the whole. For instance, leaning to cook well requires accuracy, but it also it requires flexibility and openness. You see what I mean. Macrobiotic thinking differs from modern thinking in both its ability and its willingness to look first at the whole, and only then at the parts out of which that whole is formed. If we look at life through the lens of macrobiotics, it becomes clear that each part of life is dependent on all the other parts. It follows then that if we destroy any part of life, we contribute to the destruction of all of life. On the brighter side—or what used to be called "the side of the angels"—if we enhance any part of life, we help to refresh all of life.

FOOD SECTION

RECIPES AND FOOD LISTS

SUGGESTIONS FOR GETTING STARTED

Try to use:
- Organically grown, seasonal foods where possible.
- Whole grains instead of refined grains and brown rice instead of white rice.
- Un-yeasted sourdough bread.
- One fresh vegetable dish for every meal.
- Unrefined white sea salt.
- Unrefined oils, such as light sesame oil, organic extra virgin olive oil, or safflower oil.
- Jams without added sugar.
- Fruit juices without added sugar.
- Rice syrup, maple syrup, and barley-malt syrup as natural sweeteners instead of sugar, honey, stevia, or agave nectar.
- Wild white-meat fish or salmon over meat and chicken.
- Proteins such as beans, tofu, seitan, and tempeh instead of meat and cheese.
- Non-stimulating teas and grain coffees.

- Sea vegetables for your cooking. These vegetables are sources of valuable nutrients, including calcium and beta-carotene that help reduce cholesterol, rid the body of toxins, and strengthen immunity.
- Foods from the FOODS FOR REGULAR USE list.

ABOUT CHEF SUSAN WAXMAN

Growing up in rural Pennsylvania Dutch Country, my family was always important to me. I spent a lot of time with my grandparents and extended family. When I was in my teens, some of my relatives began to develop degenerative health problems such as diabetes, high blood pressure, and cholesterol. I became concerned that the same health problems could become part of my future, since science showed that many of these health problems were hereditary. While I led a very active lifestyle throughout my high school years, college food (and beer) caught up with me, and I began to be concerned about my own health.

Over the next few years, as I watched many of my close family members struggle with health problems and making healthy lifestyle changes later in life, I decided I would rather make changes to my own lifestyle while I was young. I knew that many health problems were diet-related, so I eliminated sugar from my diet. As I became more interested in eating for health, I also became aware of the cruelty involved in raising and killing animals for daily food, and subsequently stopped eating meat.

It was around this time that I enrolled in martial-arts classes. One night after class, my sensei, Ralph, who was also a shiatsu massage practitioner, invited me to attend a lecture on macrobiotics given by his shiatsu teacher, Patrick Riley.

At this time, I was working in the social services field. I had a degree in Human Relations and was contemplating graduate school. Needless to say, going to that lecture changed my life. Macrobiotic philosophy made perfect sense to me. I liked the idea that we are all in control of our destinies. I was already eating brown rice, beans, and fresh vegetables, supplemented by the occasional miso soup, so for me to transition to the macrobiotic diet was just a matter of making a few small changes to my diet and lifestyle.

Going to this lecture was also my realization of what I wanted to do with my life. It was like a light bulb going off: I was going to study and become a macrobiotic counselor. I had known previously that I wanted to work with people, help them, and do work that is meaningful in the world.

I was already a counselor of sorts through my work in social services. I realized I would really be able to help people with their health on many different levels through macrobiotics.

Shortly after this, I began my macrobiotic studies. I started reading books by Michio Kushi and George Ohsawa. I also completed a Level I Zen shiatsu class. The next step for me was to formally study macrobiotics at the Kushi Institute. After completing my Kushi Level One studies, my teachers encouraged me to teach cooking. At this point, I didn't think I knew enough to teach, but I decided to follow their advice and taught some beginner classes from home. People seemed to enjoy my classes, and it was a great way to gain confidence and experience for what would be my eventual career.

After finishing my studies at the Kushi Institute, I began advanced studies with my future husband, Denny Waxman. I found Denny's insights into health, macrobiotics, and food to be detailed and innovative, completely broadening my understanding of macrobiotics. I thought he was brilliant. Studying with Denny was my graduate school of macrobiotics. In 1997, Denny founded The Strengthening Health Institute to train and educate teachers and counselors; I was part of the first graduating class. You might say that the rest is history, as I am currently the co-director of The Strengthening Health Institute.

I have dedicated my life to understanding the energetic nature of foods, cooking styles, and creating dynamic, healthful meal plans. All this has helped me to further develop myself as a person, my teaching, and my craft, macrobiotic cooking. Macrobiotics was one of the first things that kept my full interest; it never gets boring. As the world changes, as I change, we continuously evolve our practice of this art and way of life. I love sharing what I have learned with my students.

INTRODUCTION TO THE RECIPES
AND HEALTHFUL FOODS LIST

Welcome to the Food Section! This part of the book highlights the implementation of macrobiotic cooking from the
Strengthening Health approach. After getting into the recipes,
you'll encounter the Healthful Foods List, which places all
types of foods into categories of how often to eat them and
incorporate them into your cooking. After the recipe section,
I've included a ten-day menu plan for you to try out some of
the recipes, to monitor how you feel and look, and to have a
bit more guidance as to how to use these recipes and familiarize yourself with a macrobiotic diet.

Everybody wants to eat what I make. Cooking, for me,
is in part a constant process of learning about all aspects of
food. This helps to guide the practice of cooking into the
development of a craft, which is as varying and changing as an
individual changes. And as the craft develops, it becomes an art
form. Cooking is my art form. I enjoy using the principles
of macrobiotics in bringing a different set of techniques and
intentions into the kitchen. I like to combine the intentions

that traditional cooking uses to bring out certain aspects of flavor with the energetic principles of macrobiotic cooking. So macrobiotic cooking is both simply healthful eating and can be applied as a healing art, and I feel that with my years of practice, I've found a nice harmony between cooking daily food and healing food.

My cooking has been described as a fusion where I like to use a blend of traditional ingredients and seasonings from different cultures. I keep in mind macrobiotic principles of balance in everything I make, from the choice of ingredients to the order in which I add an ingredient or seasoning. By doing this, I have been able to merge the good flavor of my food together with dishes that have the ability to create lasting health. My ingredients are generally simple. It is my feeling that you can make great-tasting dishes while still maintaining the integrity of balance and good health.

The macrobiotic cooking and way of eating is well beyond the dieting choices of vegetarian or vegan cooking. I like to think of it as the most well thought out of the plant-based diets. Macrobiotics as a whole is really a lifestyle practice. If you want to cultivate your intuition and awareness about food, the best way to do it is to keep a simple journal after you eat and when you cook. Together with good food, a natural awakening follows, and the best part about it is that you can do it on your own.

I'm just getting started, though. There's endless variety and endless possibilities, and I could go on and on with describing combinations alone. I consider the following as a complete sampling so you can experience the realm of possibilities within macrobiotics. In my blog and cookbook to follow,

"Taste with Integrity" I plan to share more about the energetic macrobiotic principles and my interpretation of them in my cooking and seminars. I hope you enjoy these recipes and enjoy cooking and, even more so, enjoy eating them and the good health they bring to you. Thank you!

RECIPES

RECIPES

GRAINS

BREAKFAST GRAINS

There are many theories surrounding the benefits of eating breakfast. When I was growing up, my parents would often say, "start your day off right by eating a good breakfast." Many people say that breakfast is the most important meal of the day. While I don't necessarily consider breakfast to be the most important meal of the day, I do think that eating breakfast is beneficial to most people for several reasons.

Eating breakfast activates our metabolism and keeps our blood sugar stable. When our blood sugar is stable, we have better overall energy and are better able to focus throughout the morning. Breakfast does not have to be a large meal—just enough food to lightly raise your blood sugar and get your motor running will do the trick. I do think that breakfast is important for children and teenagers, because eating breakfast will help them focus in school. If you want to shed a few pounds or maintain an appropriate weight, then breakfast is very important because it will help to keep your metabolism more active throughout the day.

Note: When planning your breakfast, choose a grain-based dish and complete the meal with a light vegetable side dish, such as steamed or blanched greens.

SOFT RICE

You can easily make soft rice out of any leftover rice dish. You are simply adding water and cooking the rice until it reaches a soft and creamy consistency. I think that you will find this dish to be both nourishing and satisfying.

Preparation time: 30 minutes
Serves 2

Ingredients
- 1 cup leftover brown rice
- Water as needed, approximately 2 cups

Preparation
- Pour ½ cup of water into a pot, and begin to heat on a low flame.
- After 1 minute or so, add the rice to the pot. As the rice begins to cook it will absorb some of the water. Use a wooden spoon or rice paddle to break up any clumps of rice.
- Add a little more water and bring to a very gentle boil.
- Place a flame deflector under the pot and partially cover.
- Gently fold the bottom to the top every few minutes to prevent sticking.
- Continue to add water and cook on low until the rice is soft and creamy in texture.
- Soft rice needs to simmer 20 to 30 minutes.

Variations
- Add a little umeboshi plum toward the end of cooking. Umeboshi soft rice strengthens our digestive system and is the universal cure for flu and cold symptoms.
- Add a little of fresh or frozen corn toward the end of cooking time. This variation is helpful when trying to relax a tight condition and for prostate problems.
- When making this dish for kids, trying adding a little rice syrup or barley malt to sweeten the soft rice.

STEEL-CUT OATS

Steel-cut oats take a little more time and planning than rolled oats, but they are much more nourishing.

Preparation time: 45 to 50 minutes
Serves 4

Ingredients
- 1 cup steel-cut oats
- 4 to 5 cups water
- 1/16 teaspoon sea salt

Preparation
- Place steel-cut oats and 2 cups water in a saucepan.
- Bring the water and oats to a boil, then add the sea salt.
- Lower the flame and allow the oats to begin to absorb some of the water, about 5 to 7 minutes.
- Add another 2 cups of water and partially cover the pot. Bring the water to a boil, then lower the flame and cover. Place a flame deflector under the pot and simmer on low for 20 minutes.
- Uncover the pot, fold the bottom into the top to help the oats cook evenly and prevent them from sticking.
- Simmer another 15 minutes and serve.

Note: If you like a creamier consistency, you can add a little more water to the dish while it is simmering.

ROLLED OATS

Rolled oats come in various textures and thickness. I prefer the "thick-cut" rolled oats for their heartier texture.

Preparation time: 10 to 15 minutes
Serves 2

Ingredients
- 1 cup thick-cut rolled oats
- 2 cups water
- 1/16 teaspoon sea salt

Preparation
- Place 1½ cups of water and the oats in a pot. Let the oats sit in the water for 2 to 3 minutes.
- Turn the flame on a low setting and bring to a boil, uncovered.
- Add the sea salt.
- As the oats begin to absorb some of the water, add more water and gently fold the bottom into the top to blend the ingredients.
- Cook uncovered for a few minutes, stirring occasionally.
- As the oats continue to cook, the consistency will thicken and the texture will become more creamy. Continue to cook for another 5 minutes.
- Cover completely, turn off the flame, and let sit for another 4 to 5 minutes before serving.

SOFT MILLET

Soft millet with sweet vegetables is a very stabilizing porridge. By that, I mean it has a natural balancing effect on our blood sugar so it is helpful for both hypoglycemia and diabetes.

Preparation time: 1 hour
Serves 4 to 5

Ingredients
- 1 cup millet
- 1 cup diced onions
- ½ to 1 cup chopped sweet vegetable of your choice (carrots, winter squash, cabbage, etc.)
- 1/16 to 1/8 teaspoon sea salt
- 5 to 5½ cups water

Preparation
- Place the onions in a pot with ½ cup water and bring the water to a boil.
- Add a few grains salt and cook the onions for 2 to 3 minutes.
- Add the other vegetables, the millet, the remaining water, and the salt.
- Partially cover and bring to a boil.
- Lower the flame, cover completely, place a flame deflector under the pot, and cook for 40 minutes.
- Remove the lid and fold the top into the bottom to blend the vegetables with the millet. The texture should be creamy. Add more water as needed to reach the desired consistency.
- Replace the cover and cook for another 10 minutes.

Note: Soft millet can be made using leftover millet. Just add a little water to the bottom of a pot. Add the millet and slowly begin to heat (this is very similar to the preparation for soft rice). Add additional water as needed and continue to cook until you reach the desired consistency.

SWEET COUSCOUS

Breakfast couscous cooks very quickly and is a time-saver for busy mornings.

Preparation time: 10 minutes
Serves 2 to 3

Ingredients
- 1 cup whole-wheat couscous
- 1 cup organic apple juice
- 1⅓ cups water
- 1/16 teaspoon sea salt

Preparation
- Pour all wet ingredients into a pot and bring to a boil.
- Add the couscous and a pinch of salt.
- Lower the flame, cover, and place a flame deflector under the pot.
- Cook for 1 to 2 minutes on a low flame.
- Turn off the flame and let the pot sit for 5–7 minutes.
- Remove the cover and stir the couscous with a wooden spoon before serving.

STEAMED SOURDOUGH BREAD

Bread is a staple among all European cultures. Good-quality bread is satisfying, nourishing, and a good source of protein. When shopping for bread, read the ingredient label. There should only be a few main ingredients; flour, salt, and water. Real sourdough bread does not contain any yeast. Steaming bread makes the bread more digestible and makes the nutrients in the bread more bio-available.

Preparation time: 2 to 4 minutes
1 to 2 slices per person

Ingredients
- Sourdough bread
- A small amount of water for steaming
- A stainless-steel pot and a steamer basket. I prefer using a steamer basket that sits on top of the pot (not the collapsible ones that fit inside). You can use either a stainless-steel or bamboo steamer basket; both work well.

Preparation
- Add an inch of water to cover the bottom of the pot and place the steamer basket on top of the pot.
- Place the bread inside the basket, turn on the flame, and cover.
- When the bread gives off a "fresh-baked" aroma, after 2–5 minutes, it is ready.
- Remove the bread from the basket, place it on a bamboo mat that is on top of a plate.
- Allow the bread to cool a bit before adding your favorite topping.

Topping Suggestions: Tahini or peanut butter and sauerkraut, tahini or peanut butter and fruit spread, hummus and sauerkraut with cucumbers, onion, or squash butter.

OTHER GRAINS

BROWN RICE

As the most balanced of all cereal grains, brown rice has many unique qualities. Unlike other grains, it grows on both dry land and in water. Brown rice is also very flexible and adaptable in that it combines well with other grains, beans, and vegetables. Of all the whole-cereal grains, brown rice has the greatest ability to bring our bodies into balance and strengthen our overall health.

Despite its numerous benefits, it is possible to eat too much brown rice! For most people, a serving of brown rice 5 to 7 days a week is enough to create a good condition and maintain strong vitality. Eating too much brown rice creates an overly contracted internal condition which can lead to other health problems. Personally, I like to combine my brown rice with other grains and beans. This combination gives us strength and vitality while also providing more variety in our diet. Below is a recipe for basic brown rice and some helpful hints on how to prepare rice combinations, including how to vary the proportions to create a balance that suits your personal needs.

PRESSURE-COOKED BROWN RICE WITH GRAINS

Preparation time: 50 to 60 minutes
2 cups of dry brown rice yields 5 to 6 servings

Ingredients
- 1⅔ cups organic brown rice
- ⅓ cup grain, such as sweet brown rice or barley
- 2½ to 2⅔ cups water
- ⅛ teaspoon sea salt or 1 square inch kombu

Preparation
- Wash the rice by placing it in a bowl and covering with water. Use your hand to gently swish the grain around several times, then pour the water off. Repeat this process two more times, for a total of three rinses.
- Whole grains may be washed and soaked together with the brown rice.
- Partially refined (pearled) or cracked grains are not soaked and are added right before you are ready to cook your rice.
- Place washed grain in a bowl along with the pre-measured water to soak. Soaking the rice makes it more digestible, allowing the grain to open up and release more nutrients. I recommend soaking rice overnight, up to 20 hours.
- Place the rice and the soaking water in a pressure cooker.
- Add the sea salt or kombu, cover, and bring to full pressure on a medium flame.
- Place a flame deflector under the pressure cooker and reduce the flame to low.
- Cook under low pressure for 45 to 50 minutes.
- Turn off the flame and remove pot from the stove.
- Let sit, allowing the pressure to come down naturally.

- Remove the rice from the pressure cooker using a moistened wooden rice paddle.
- Place the rice in a bowl and cover with a light bamboo mat until ready to serve.

POT-BOILED BROWN RICE

I like to boil my rice in warmer weather, since boiling is a lighter style of cooking than pressure-cooking. I sometimes choose to cook a 50/50 combination of brown rice together with another grain to produce an even lighter energetic effect. Be sure to use a sturdy pot with a heavy lid when boiling brown rice so that moisture does not escape.

Preparation time: 65 to 70 minutes
Serves 4 to 5

Ingredients
- 1 cup brown rice
- 2 cups water

Preparation
- Place the soaked rice and soaking water in a pot.
- If you are adding any partially refined or cracked grain, add it at this time along with any additional water needed to keep the 1:2 grain-to-water ratio.
- Bring the water to a boil over a medium-high flame.
- When the water begins to boil add a small pinch of sea salt or kombu sea vegetable.
- Cover, place a flame deflector under the pot and reduce the heat to the lowest setting.

- Simmer on low for 1 hour.
- Remove the the rice using a moistened wooden paddle and place the rice in a serving bowl. Cover the rice with a bamboo mat until serving time.

Favorite Brown Rice and Grain Combinations
Pearled barley
Hato mugi barley
Farro
Cracked wheat
Sweet brown rice
Quinoa
Rye

VEGETABLE FRIED RICE

Fried rice is a rich and satisfying dish that works best using leftover rice.

Preparation time: 10 to 15 minutes
Serves 4

Ingredients
- 1½ cups leftover rice
- ⅓ cup carrot, diced
- ½ cup onion, diced
- ⅓ cup scallion, diced into ¼-inch-thick pieces
- ¹⁄₁₆ to ⅛ teaspoon sea salt
- ¾ to 1 teaspoon shoyu
- Fresh ginger juice, to taste
- 1 tablespoon light sesame oil or olive oil
- ½ cup water

Variations

- Use thin slices of snow peas or edamame in place of the scallion.
- Use only one vegetable, such as spring onions or scallions.
- Add sliced mushrooms for a rich, earthy taste.
- Black or red pepper may be used for additional seasoning.

Preparation

- Pour the oil in a cast-iron wok or stainless-steel skillet and gently heat over a low flame.
- Add the onion and begin sautéeing. When the onions begin to glisten, add a tiny pinch of sea salt and continue to sautée.
- Add a little water to moisten the skillet, then add the carrots.
- Continue to sautée for 2 to 3 minutes for an al dente texture. For a softer texture, cover and simmer the vegetables for another 2 to 3 minutes.
- Add the scallions and combine with the other vegetables.
- Season lightly with 3 or 4 drops of the shoyu and gently fold the vegetable mixture over to blend the seasoning.
- Reduce the flame, add a little more water to the bottom of the pan, then add the rice.
- Place a cover on the pot and simmer for 1 to 2 minutes to allow the rice to soften.
- Lightly season with the remainder of the shoyu and blend well with the rice and vegetables. At the very end of cooking, add the fresh grated ginger juice or pepper.
- Place the rice in a serving bowl and cover with a bamboo mat.

FRIED RICE WITH FRESH HERBS
AND VEGETABLES

This is a lighter, more refreshing version of my traditional vegetable fried rice.

Preparation time: 10 minutes
Serves 4

Ingredients
- 1½ cups cooked medium or long-grain rice
- 1 cup red onion, sliced in ⅛-inch-thick half moons
- ½ cup thinly sliced leek
- 1 to 2 tablespoons light sesame or olive oil
- ¼ to ⅓ cup chopped cilantro or fresh parsley, stems removed
- ⅛ to ¼ teaspoon sea salt
- Dash umeboshi vinegar
- Fresh-squeezed lemon or lime juice
- Water
- Toasted sunflower seeds, optional garnish

Preparation
- Pour the oil in a cast-iron wok or stainless-steel skillet and gently heat over a low flame.
- Add the onions to the skillet and sauté. If the pan becomes dry, add a small amount of water to the skillet to moisten the onions.
- When the onions are evenly coated with oil, add a pinch of salt and a splash of umeboshi vinegar.
- Add the leeks and continue to sauté the vegetables until they reach the desired texture. I prefer to keep them on the crunchier side for this dish.
- Add a little more water to moisten the pan and the leftover rice.

- Gently fold the vegetables into the rice using a wooden spatula.
- Lightly season the rice with a few drops of umeboshi vinegar.
- Turn off the flame and add the chopped fresh herbs and fresh-squeezed lime juice to taste.
- Use the spatula to gently blend all the ingredients.
- Place the rice in a serving bowl and cover with a bamboo mat until serving time.

MILLET WITH SWEET VEGETABLES

Millet is a whole grain that is helpful for upper-body problems. It is very balancing for the central organs and good for stabilizing the blood sugar.

Preparation time: 1 hour
Serves: 4 to 5

Ingredients
- 1 cup millet
- ½ cup diced onions
- ⅔ cups diced sweet vegetables, such as cabbage, carrots, or squash
- 3¼ to 4 cups water
- 1/16 teaspoon sea salt

Preparation
- Place the millet in a bowl and examine to check for any small pebbles or unwanted debris, then rinse until the water is clear and set aside.
- Place the onions on the bottom of the pot with just enough water to cover and bring to a boil. Add a tiny pinch of sea

salt (just a few grains) and cook 5 minutes or until the water begins to evaporate.
- Layer any round vegetables (such as cabbage) you are using on top of the onions, followed by any root vegetables, then the millet.
- Add the remaining water and a tiny pinch of sea salt.
- Cover and bring to a boil on a medium flame.
- Place a flame deflector underneath the pot and simmer on low for 40 minutes.
- Remove the grain from the pot, place in serving dish, and cover with a sushi mat until serving.

Favorite Vegetable Combinations
Onion, cabbage, carrot
Onion, cauliflower
Onion, leeks, parsnips
Onion, sweet potato
Onion, cabbage, parsnip
Onion, leeks, carrots

BARLEY BEAN STEW

Preparation time: 1½ hours
Serves 4 to 6

Ingredients
- 1 cup pearled barley, washed
- 1 cup precooked white beans with ⅓ cup of their cooking liquid. Organic canned beans work well too, as does fried tempeh.

- 1½ cups diced onions
- 1 cup diced root vegetables. Choose one or a combination of carrots and/or parsnips.
- 1 cup diced leeks or celery
- ½ to ¾ teaspoon sea salt
- 2¼ cups water
- 1 to 2 tablespoons olive oil or light sesame oil

Preparation
- Place the onion in a pot with ¼ cup of water.
- Turn on the flame and begin to cook the onions. When the onions begin to glisten, add a small pinch of sea salt (about ¹⁄₁₆ teaspoon).
- Allow the onions to cook on their own for 3 to 5 minutes.
- Layer the leeks and celery on top of the onions, followed by the root vegetables and pearled barley.
- Add additional water and bring to a boil.
- Add another ⅛ teaspoon sea salt, cover, and place a flame deflector under the pot.
- Lower the flame and simmer on low for 30 minutes.
- Add the white beans and the remaining salt. Gently fold the beans into the stew to blend the ingredients and the seasoning. Cook for another 20 minutes.

For a richer flavor, sautée ½ cup diced onions and/or leeks together with the white beans, then mix to combine with the barley and vegetables.

PERUVIAN QUINOA WITH BLACK BEANS AND AVOCADO

Preparation time: 45 minutes to 1 hour
Serves 4

Ingredients
- 1 cup white quinoa, or a mixture of white and red quinoa
- 1¾ cups water
- 1/16 teaspoon sea salt for cooking the quinoa
- 1 cup diced red onion
- 2½ to 3 tablespoons olive oil
- 1½ cups pre-cooked black or red beans
- ½ to ¾ teaspoon sea salt
- 2¼ teaspoons umeboshi vinegar
- ⅓ to ½ cup chopped cilantro
- 1 avocado, diced
- Fresh-squeezed lime juice, to taste
- Red chili or jalapeño pepper, seeds removed and finely sliced, optional

Preparation
- Place the quinoa and 1¾ cups water in a pot and bring to a boil.
- Add a small pinch of sea salt, cover, and place a flame deflector under the pot.
- Lower the flame and simmer on low for 15 minutes.
- Remove the quinoa from the pot, place in a bowl, and set aside.
- Heat the olive oil in a separate pan.
- Add the red onions and begin to sautée.
- When the onions begin to glisten, add a small pinch of sea salt, ¼ cup water, and continue to sautée.

- Add the black beans and a small amount of bean cooking liquid, to keep the mixture moist.
- Add the remaining sea salt and fold to blend the seasoning.
- Lower the flame and let simmer 6 to 7 minutes.
- Turn off the flame, then add the cooked quinoa.
- Drizzle 1 tablespoon olive oil over the grain.
- Add half the chopped cilantro, the avocado, and a little fresh-squeezed lime juice.
- Gently fold to mix all the ingredients together.
- Place in a serving dish and garnish with a little freshly made guacamole if desired.

BULGUR WHEAT SALAD

Preparation time: 45 minutes
Serves 2 to 4

Ingredients
- ½ cup bulgur wheat or quinoa for a gluten-free version
- 1 cup water
- Pinch sea salt
- ½ cup diced red onion (raw or lightly blanched)
- ½ cup chopped cucumber
- ½ to ⅓ cup finely chopped parsley
- 2 to 2½ tablespoons olive oil
- ¼ to ½ teaspoon sea salt
- ¼ to ½ teaspoon umeboshi vinegar
- 1½ to 2 tablespoons fresh-squeezed lemon juice
- ⅓ cup chopped tomatoes, optional

Preparation

- Place the onion and cucumber in a bowl.
- Add a small pinch of sea salt and use your hands to gently mix the salt with the vegetables.
- Put a small plate over the vegetables to lightly press them. Set vegetables aside while you cook the bulgur.
- Place bulgur and water in a pan, turn on the flame, and bring to a boil.
- Add ¼ teaspoon sea salt. Cover, reduce heat to low, place a flame deflector under the pot, and cook for 20 minutes.
- Immediately remove the bulgur from the pot and place in a serving dish. Use a wooden utensil moistened with olive oil to gently fluff the grain and get rid of any clumps.
- Remove the plate from the diced vegetables, and pour off any liquid.
- Add the parsley to the vegetables, then the olive oil and umeboshi vinegar, and combine.
- Add the vegetables to the warm bulgur, together with a squeeze of fresh lemon.
- Gently mix with a wooden utensil to thoroughly blend all the ingredients.

POLENTA

Preparation time: 50 minutes to 1 hour
Serves 4

Ingredients
- 1 cup corn grits or polenta
- 5 cups water
- ¼ to ½ teaspoon sea salt
- 1 to 1½ tablespoons extra virgin olive oil, optional

Preparation
- Pour 4 cups water in a pot and begin to heat over a medium-high flame.
- Just before the water comes to a full boil, add the sea salt and begin to sift the cornmeal into the pot. This was traditionally done by using one hand as a funnel, while constantly stirring with the other hand. Stirring is very important to prevent clumping!
- Gradually add the remaining water, a little at a time.
- Continue this method until all the grain is used.
- Add the olive oil, if using, and continue stirring to blend the oil with the grain.
- Continue stirring until the polenta is thick and creamy.
- Lower the flame and place a flame deflector under the pot, cover and simmer on the lowest setting for 30 minutes.
- Serve immediately, or pour the hot polenta into a flat pyrex pan. As the polenta cools, it will firm up and set. You can serve firm polenta at room temperature, or you can steam, pan-fry, or grill it.

COUSCOUS VEGETABLE SALAD WITH RED ONION, CARROT, AND PEAS

Preparation time: 45 minutes
Serves 2 to 4

Ingredients
- 1 cup couscous
- 2 cups water
- ⅓ cup carrot, diced
- ⅓ cup green peas
- ½ cup red onion, diced
- ⅓ cup finely chopped parsley
- 1½ tablespoons extra virgin olive oil
- ¼ teaspoon toasted sesame oil
- ⅛ teaspoon sea salt
- 1½ to 2 teaspoons shoyu
- 2 to 2½ teaspoons umeboshi vinegar
- black pepper (optional)

Preparation
- Place the water and sea salt in a pot and bring to a boil.
- Place couscous in a bowl.
- Pour the boiling water over the couscous.
- Cover the bowl and let sit for 5 minutes, or 8 minutes when using whole-wheat couscous.
- Rub a little olive oil on your hands or use an oiled wooden spatula to break up any lumps and fluff the couscous.
- Cover couscous with a mat and set aside while you cook the vegetables.
- Gently heat a few drops of oil in a skillet, then add the onion and sautée.

- When the onion begins to glisten, add a pinch of salt and a little water.
- Add the carrots and continue to sautée. Cover and simmer for 2 to 3 minutes.
- Season the vegetables with shoyu.
- Add the green peas, turn off the flame, and gently fold to mix all of the vegetables.
- Add the couscous, a drizzle of olive oil, and the chopped parsley.
- Gently fold to mix all ingredients.
- Add the umeboshi vinegar and a little black pepper if using, and fold to blend the seasonings.
- Place in a bowl and cover with a mat until you are ready to serve.

Variations
- Substitute cooked chickpeas for the green peas.
- Add seitan or fried tempeh for a heartier dish.

FARRO WITH WHITE BEANS AND KALE

Preparation time: 1 hour
Serves 2 to 4

Ingredients
- 1 cup farro
- 2 cups water
- 1 cup diced onions
- 1 cup pre-cooked white beans
- ½ cup finely chopped kale

- ¼ cup extra virgin olive oil
- ¾ to 1 teaspoon sea salt
- sliced or whole garlic cloves, optional
- black or red pepper flakes, optional

Preparation

- Place farro and water in a pot and bring to a boil.
- Add a small pinch of sea salt.
- Cover, place a flame deflector under the pot, and simmer on low heat for 35 to 40 minutes.
- Pour enough olive oil into a separate pan to coat the bottom. Turn on the flame and begin to heat the oil.
- Add the onions and begin to sautée.
- Add a few tablespoons water, ⅛ teaspoon sea salt, and continue to sautée. Add the garlic and/or red pepper flakes if you are using them.
- Add the white beans and a little of the bean juice.
- Add additional sea salt and continue to simmer over a medium-low flame for 10 minutes.
- Add the chopped kale, fold to blend all the ingredients together. Simmer for another 7 to 10 minutes.
- Use a wooden utensil and add the farro to the vegetables and beans. Gently fold to blend the ingredients.
- For additional richness and flavor, drizzle a little olive oil over the grain and add another small pinch of sea salt, about ⅛ teaspoon. Add black pepper if using.
- Fold to blend all the ingredients.
- Place the farro in a serving bowl and cover with a bamboo mat until ready to serve.

⊰◈⊱

SAFFRON RISOTTO

Preparation time: 1 hour
Serves 4

Ingredients
- 2 cups risotto rice
- 1½ tablespoons olive oil
- 1 to 2 cloves of garlic, peeled and cut in half lengthwise
- A splash of white wine, approximately ⅛ cup
- 1 cup diced onion
- 1 cup diced carrot
- ½ cup green peas
- 2 quarts vegetable stock
- ¾ to 1 teaspoon sea salt
- A few strands of saffron (⅛ to ¼ teaspoon)
- Cracked black pepper to taste, optional

Variations
- Use chopped asparagus or green beans in place of the peas.
- Add additional summer vegetables, such as yellow squash or zucchini.

Preparation
- Heat the olive oil in a pot over low heat.
- Add onion and begin to sautée until the onions begin to glisten, then add the garlic and a pinch of sea salt. Continue to sautée.
- Add the rice and sautée until the rice is evenly coated with the oil-and-onion mixture.
- Add white wine to just cover the rice. When the wine is absorbed, add ¼ cup stock. Gently stir after adding the

stuck to prevent the rice from sticking. Once the rice has absorbed the stock, add the saffron and carrots and additional sea salt at this time. Gently fold all ingredients together.

- Continue adding the stock in small increments, about ¼ to ½ cup at a time and folding until you are close to reaching the texture you desire. This takes approximately 25 to 35 minutes.
- Add the peas near the end of cooking and mix throughout the risotto.
- Add black pepper and a drizzle of olive oil to finish off the dish.

NOODLES AND PASTA SAUCES

UDON NOODLES WITH SAUTÉED VEGETABLES

Preparation time: 30 minutes
Serves 3 to 4

Ingredients
- 1½ cups water
- ½ teaspoon toasted sesame oil
- 1 tablespoon light sesame oil or 2 tablespoons olive oil
- 1 pack pre-cooked udon noodles
- 1½ cup onions, sliced into ¼-inch half-moons
- ½ cup carrots, cut into thin matchsticks
- 3 to 4 stalks of bok choy, cut on the angle, stems removed from the leaves
- ¾ teaspoon sea salt
- ¼ to ½ teaspoon shoyu
- Fresh grated ginger juice and/or shichimi, optional

Preparation
- Gently heat the oil in a deep pan or wok.
- Add the onions and begin to sautée.
- Add a little water and ¼ tsp. sea salt and continue to sautée.

- Add the carrots and additional water and the rest of the salt. Cover and simmer for 3 to 5 minutes.
- Add the bok choy bottoms and sautée for a minute, then add the bok choy leaves.
- Add the udon and the shoyu.
- Add the spice, if using.
- Gently fold to blend all the ingredients and seasonings together.

PASTA SAUCES

Note: Heat the water for the pasta so it is ready to go while you make the sauce. The cooking time will depend on what type of pasta you use. Try to time it so that the pasta will be done at the same time that you finish the sauce. If you are mixing the pasta directly in with the sauce, undercook the pasta slightly, as it will continue to cook when it is mixed with the sauce.

ONIONS, KALE, AND SUN-DRIED TOMATO SAUCE

Preparation time: 30 to 40 minutes
Sauce makes approximately 4 servings
½ package of pasta serves 2

Ingredients
- 2 cups diced onion
- ½ cup sun-dried tomatoes, reconstituted in 1 cup of water
- 3 to 5 leaves kale, chopped. Use more kale if desired.
- 1 to 2 cloves garlic
- A dash of white wine, approximately 2 ounces

- 3 to 4 tablespoons extra virgin olive oil
- 1 to 1½ teaspoons sea salt
- 1½ to 2 cups water
- Black pepper or red chili pepper to taste
- Toasted sourdough bread crumbs

Preparation
- Heat 3 tablespoons of olive oil in a saucepan.
- Add the onions and begin to sautée. Add a little bit of water to prevent the oil from getting too hot. Add ⅛ teaspoon sea salt and continue to sautée.
- Add the garlic and a splash of white wine and continue to sautée.
- Add the sun-dried tomatoes, including their soaking liquid.
- Add the kale, additional water, and more salt. Cover the pot, lower the flame, and allow to simmer for few minutes.
- Add a little black pepper and a drizzle of olive oil.
- Cook pasta al dente and toss the pasta with the vegetables and sauce.
- Add a little fried bread crumbs to each individual dish.

Variations:
- Add black olives to the sauce.

CAULIFLOWER AND BABY ARUGULA SAUCE

Preparation time: 30 to 40 minutes
Sauce makes approximately 4 servings
½ package of pasta serves 2

Ingredients
- 2 cups diced onions

- ½ head of cauliflower, cut into bite-size florets, approximately 2½ to 3 cups
- ½ to 1 cup finely grated carrot
- 2 cups baby arugula
- 2 to 3 tablespoons extra virgin olive oil
- 3 to 4 cups water
- 1½ to 2 teaspoons sea salt
- Black pepper and or red pepper
- 1 to 2 cloves of garlic, optional

Preparation

- Gently heat a small amount of olive oil in a pan.
- Add the onions and begin to sautée.
- Add a small amount of water, garlic, and a nice pinch of sea salt.
- Add the cauliflower florets, cover, and simmer for 5 to 8 minutes.
- Add some of the pasta cooking liquid and a little more salt.
- Add the grated carrot.
- Add the baby arugula.
- Add additional olive oil and a little pepper.
- Add a little fresh-squeezed lemon.
- Serve hot over pasta.

BROCCOLI AND WHITE BEANS

Preparation time: 30 to 40 minutes
Sauce makes approximately 4 to 6 servings
1 package of pasta serves 4

Ingredients

- 1½ cups diced onion
- 1 bunch of broccoli, florets separated and stems peeled
- ½ to 1 cup cooked cannellini beans
- 1 cup cherry tomatoes, cut in half, optional
- 1 to 2 cloves garlic, thinly sliced or left whole
- 5 to 6 tablespoons extra virgin olive oil
- 3 to 4 cups of liquid; use a combination of water and liquid from the cooked pasta
- 2 to 3 teaspoons sea salt
- White wine
- Red and/or black pepper, optional

Preparation

- Gently heat the olive oil in a pan.
- Add the onions and begin to sautée.
- Add a small amount of white wine and garlic. Continue to sautée.
- Add a little bit of water and the broccoli stems, cover, and simmer for 1 minute.
- Add the white beans and sea salt. Cover and simmer on low heat for another 3 minutes.
- Add the broccoli florets and additional water from the pasta cooking liquid. If you like a brothier sauce, add more liquid. Add a little more salt, cover, and simmer for 2 to 3 minutes.
- Add the cherry tomatoes, a drizzle of olive oil, additional salt if needed, and a crack of black pepper.
- Simmer uncovered for a few minutes so that the salt blends in with the other ingredients.
- Serve over pasta or add pasta directly to the sauce.

SOUPS

Soups are an important part of a healthful diet. Both strengthening and balancing, aim to have one serving of vegetable soup per day. There are two main categories of soup: savory and sweet. Both savory soups and sweet soups are delicious and healthful, although the health benefits are different for each.

Savory soups activate the digestive system and build healthy intestinal flora, helping clean out our intestines. Savory soups are seasoned with miso, sea salt, or a combination of salt and shoyu. Miso soup is the most commonly consumed savory soup in the macrobiotic diet. In addition to its delicious taste, miso is also a wonderful probiotic. Miso soup can be enjoyed 5 to 7 times per week.

Sweet soups are mildly sweet, and are often creamy in texture. The sweetness and consistency are derived by using a combination of cooked sweet vegetables. Sweet vegetables relax the central organs, which has a stabilizing effect on our blood sugar. Sweet vegetable soups are also very soothing, with their satisfying, nourishing texture. We recommend using only sea salt for seasoning sweet vegetable soups. Enjoy sweet vegetable soup about two times per week.

BASIC MISO SOUP

Miso soup strengthens and activates our digestive systems. Miso helps clean the intestinal villi and creates healthy bacteria and enzymes in the digestive tract. Enjoying miso soup regularly strengthens our digestion and alkalizes our overall condition. Note that miso soup is meant to be broth-y, so be conservative when deciding how many vegetables to add!

Preparation time: 10 minutes

Ingredients
- Wakame sea vegetable, 1 to 2 inches wakame per cup of water
- 2 to 4 thin slices of root or round vegetables per cup of water
- ⅛ to ¼ cup leafy greens, finely chopped
- Miso, use ½ to 1 level teaspoon miso per 1 cup water. Be sure to buy your miso from a reputable health-food store. Barley miso, brown rice miso, and sweet-tasting brown rice miso are all excellent options.
- 1 cup water per serving, plus an additional ⅛ cup (for two servings, measure out 2⅛ cups water)
- Scallion, finely chopped for garnish

Preparation
- Soak the wakame in water for one to two minutes, or until it is soft enough to cut. Discard the soaking water and cut the wakame into even pieces.
- Measure the water and pour into a stainless-steel pot. Place the wakame in the pot, turn on the flame, and bring to a boil.
- Add the root and/or round vegetables and cook for 4 to 5 minutes.
- While the vegetables are cooking, measure out the miso into a small bowl. Take a small ladle of the stock and use a wooden utensil to dilute the miso with the ladleful of

stock. The resulting consistency should be thin enough that it will easily dissolve when added back to the pot.
- Add the leafy greens to the pot, then add the diluted miso to the boiling water.
- Turn your flame on its lowest setting and simmer for 3 to 4 minutes.
- Place a ladle full of soup in a small bowl, garnish with finely chopped scallions, and serve.

DAIKON AND DRIED SHIITAKE MISO SOUP

Daikon and dried shiitake miso soup dissolves fat and softens hardness in the intestines. It is also good for lowering cholesterol and losing weight.

Preparation time: 10 to 15 minutes

Ingredients
- Wakame sea vegetable, use 1 to 2 inches per cup of water
- 2 to 3 pieces thinly sliced daikon radish per cup of water
- 1 to 2 dried shiitake mushrooms, soaked and thinly sliced
- ⅛ to ¼ cup leafy greens, finely chopped
- ½ to 1 level teaspoon miso per cup of water
- 1 cup water per serving, plus an additional ⅛ cup (for two servings, measure out 2⅛ cups water)
- Scallions, finely chopped for garnish

Preparation
- Soak the wakame in water for one to two minutes or until it is soft. Discard the soaking water and cut the wakame into equal pieces.

- Measure the water for the total number of servings you want, including the shiitake soaking water. Pour the liquid into a pot, add the wakame and the shiitake, and bring to a boil over a medium flame.
- Add the daikon and cook for 4 to 5 minutes.
- Measure the miso and place in a small bowl. Add a little stock and use a wooden utensil to dissolve the miso.
- Add the leafy greens to the pot, then add the diluted miso to the boiling both. Immediately lower the flame and simmer for 3 to 4 minutes. Garnish with finely chopped scallions and serve.

CREAM OF BROCCOLI SOUP

Preparation time: 45 minutes
Serves 6–7

Ingredients
- 2½ cups onions, diced
- ½ cup leek, diced
- 3 heads broccoli, stems peeled and diced, flower-cut into florets and placed in a separate bowl
- 1 cup cauliflower, cut into florets
- 7 cups water
- 1 teaspoon sea salt
- Herbs (parsley, cilantro, thyme, etc.), finely chopped for garnish

Preparation
- Place the onions and 2 cups of the water in a stock pot and bring to a boil.
- Add ⅛ teaspoon of sea salt and boil the onions for 3 to 4 minutes.

- Add the leeks, then the cauliflower and the broccoli stems.
- Add the remaining 5 cups water and the rest of the salt. Cover and bring to a boil.
- Lower the flame and simmer for 15 minutes.
- Add the broccoli florets, cover, and simmer another 5 to 7 minutes.
- Remove the pot from the stove and use an immersion blender to purée the soup.
- Garnish with your favorite fresh herbs

Variations
- For a richer taste, sautée thin slices of leek and add them to the soup. The leeks add a new dimension of flavor and are also pleasing to the eye.

CAULIFLOWER AND LEEK SOUP

Preparation time: 45 minutes
Serves 4 to 6

Ingredients
- 3 cups onions, diced
- ½ cup leeks, diced
- ½ to 1 head cauliflower, about 5–6 cups chopped florets
- 5 to 6 cups water
- ¾ teaspoon sea salt
- Parsley, finely chopped for garnish

Preparation
- Place diced onions in a pot with 1 cup water, just enough to cover the onions by an inch.

- Turn on the flame and bring to a boil.
- Add a pinch of sea salt and continue to cook the onions for several minutes or until they become translucent.
- Add the leeks, cauliflower, and enough additional water to cover the vegetables by an inch.
- Add a generous pinch of sea salt, cover, and bring to a boil on a medium-high flame.
- When water begins to boil, cover, and simmer on medium-low heat for approximately 20 minutes or until the vegetables are tender.
- Use a hand food mill or an immersion blender to purée until smooth and creamy in texture.
- Place in a serving bowl and garnish with finely chopped parsley.

Note: You can adjust the consistency by increasing or decreasing the amount of vegetables and water. If soup becomes too thick, add additional water until desired consistency is reached.

SWEET POTATO SOUP WITH CARROTS AND GINGER

Preparation time: 40 minutes
Serves 5 to 6 people

Ingredients
- 3 cups diced onion
- 4 cups sweet potato, peeled and cut into 1-inch cubes
- 2 cups diced carrot

- 5 to 6 cups water
- ¾ to 1 teaspoon sea salt
- 1-inch knob fresh ginger, grated and juice reserved
- Garnish options: fried tarragon, minced parsley, fried parsley

Preparation
- Place the onions in a pot with 1½ cups of the water. Bring to a boil, then add ⅛ teaspoon sea salt, reduce the flame to medium-low, and simmer uncovered for 5 minutes.
- Add the sweet potato and the carrots.
- Add the rest of the water and ¾ teaspoon salt. Cover and bring to a boil.
- Reduce the flame and simmer on low for 20 minutes or until the vegetables are soft.
- Remove from the stove and purée with an immersion blender until smooth and velvety. Grate the ginger using a fine ginger grater, then squeeze the juice into the soup, stirring to incorporate.
- Place in individual serving bowls and garnish with your favorite choice of fresh herbs.

RED BEAN SOUP

Preparation time: 45 minutes
Serves 4 to 6

Ingredients
- 3 to 4 cups cooked red beans or kidney beans, reserving the cooking liquid
- 3 cups diced onion

- ¾ cup diced celery
- 1 cup diced carrot
- ½ cup leek or scallion, thinly sliced
- 6 to 7 cups water
- 2½ teaspoons sea salt

For sautéed vegetables:
- 1 cup diced onion
- ½ cup leek and/or scallion, thinly sliced
- 1 teaspoon olive oil
- 1 teaspoon toasted sesame oil
- Fresh cilantro or Italian parsley, finely chopped
- Optional: black and/or red pepper, thinly sliced fresh garlic

Preparation
- Place the onions and 3 cups of the water in a stock pot and bring to a boil.
- Add ⅛ teaspoon sea salt, lower the flame, and simmer the onions for 3 minutes.
- Add the celery and simmer another minute. If using the garlic, add it at this time.
- Add the carrot, beans, additional water, and sea salt.
- Cover and bring to a boil. Lower the flame, place a flame deflector under the pot, and simmer 15 minutes.
- While the soup is simmering, prepare the sautéed vegetables.
- Gently heat the toasted sesame and olive oils in a skillet.
- Add the onions and begin to sautée. When the onions begin to sweat, add a small pinch of sea salt and a scant ¼ cup water. Cook until the onions are translucent.
- Add the leeks and/or the scallions, and continue to sautée. Add more water as needed to keep the pan moist. When the vegetables are soft, add them to the soup pot.
- Add another ½ teaspoon of sea salt, cover, and simmer for another 10 minutes.

- Add the pepper and the fresh herbs. Simmer uncovered for another 5 minutes.
- Serve hot and garnish with the finely chopped fresh herbs.

SPLIT PEA SOUP

This soup is so popular that I always have to make extra, so this recipe makes a large quantity of soup. You can always make half of the amount or freeze some for a later day.

Preparation time: 3 hours
Serves 8–10

Ingredients
- 4 cups split peas
- 4½ cups diced onion
- 1 cup diced leek
- ½ cup finely diced burdock
- 10 to 12 cups water
- 2½-inch strip kombu sea vegetable, rinsed
- 2 tablespoons sea salt
- 1 teaspoon shoyu
- Black and/or red pepper, to taste
- Fresh herbs (I like parsley or sweet basil), finely chopped
- Optional: a splash of red wine and a drizzle of olive oil and/ or deep-fried sourdough croutons

Preparation
- Place the onions and 4 cups of the water in a deep stock pot. Split peas foam during the initial cooking, so using a deeper pot will prevent a huge mess on your stove.

- Bring the water to a boil and cook the onions for 4 minutes.
- Add the leek, then the burdock.
- Layer the peas on top of the vegetables.
- Add 6 cups of water and bring to a boil, uncovered.
- Skim off any excess foam, lower the flame to a relaxed rolling boil, and continue to cook uncovered until the foaming diminishes.
- Place a flame deflector under the pot, cover and lower the flame.
- Simmer on low for 1½ hours. Check the peas and use a wooden spoon to stir the soup.
- Cover and continue to cook until the peas are completely soft, about 2 hours.
- Add the salt and stir with a wooden spoon. Cover and simmer for 15 minutes.
- Add any additional water to reach the desired consistency.
- Add the shoyu, pepper, and any of the optional ingredients.
- Simmer for another 5 minutes, then garnish with the fresh herbs and serve.

PURÉED CHICKPEA SOUP

Preparation time: 2 hours
Serves 5 to 6

Ingredients
- 1½ cups chickpeas or white beans, soaked 6 to 8 hours
- 4 cups diced onions
- 6 cups water
- 1-inch piece kombu sea vegetable, rinsed
- 1½ teaspoons sea salt

- Fresh herbs such as sweet basil, thyme, or oregano; choose one fresh herb or a combination of herbs
- Fresh lemon juice; 1-inch-thick wedge or slightly more
- Black pepper to taste

Cookware
- 3.5 liter pressure cooker
- Long-handled wooden spoon
- Immersion blender

Preparation
- Rinse and soak the dry beans 6 to 8 hours or overnight.
- Discard the bean soaking water, add some fresh water, and rinse the beans.
- Place the diced onions in a pressure cooker add enough water to cover (2 cups).
- Bring the water to a boil, then add the kombu.
- Lower the flame and cook the onions for 4 to 5 minutes.
- Add the soaked beans and the remaining water.
- Bring the water to a boil. Skim off any foam that rises.
- Place the lid on the pressure cooker and bring to full pressure.
- Place a flame deflector under the pot, reduce the flame, and pressure cook for 50 to 60 minutes (if using cannellini beans, cook for 30 minutes).
- Remove the pot from the stove, take the pressure down, and remove lid.
- Return the pot to the stove and turn the flame on low.
- Add the sea salt, bring to a light boil, and simmer for 10 minutes.
- Turn off the flame and use a hand immersion blender to purée the soup.
- Return the pot to the stove, then add the fresh herbs.
- Garnish with a drizzle of olive oil, fresh herbs, and black pepper to individual taste.

CLEAR SOUP

Preparation time: 30 minutes
Serves 4 to 6

Ingredients
- 1 medium-large dried shiitake mushroom
- 2-to-4 inch strip kombu
- 6 cups water
- ¾ teaspoon sea salt
- ½ cup onions, cut into thin half-moons
- 5 drops shoyu, about ⅛ teaspoon
- 3 pieces konyaku bows per bowl of soup
- 2 pieces fried mochi or fresh tofu per bowl of soup
- A small amount of baby kale to garnish each bowl

Soup Preparation
- Place the water in a pot together with the kombu and dried shiitake.
- Bring the water to a boil, then lower the flame to a rolling boil and continue cooking for 2 to 3 minutes.
- Remove the kombu and shiitake.
- Add the onions and a small pinch of salt.
- Slice the dried shiitake and return it to the pot.
- Add the remaining ¼ teaspoon sea salt, reduce the flame, and simmer for another 5 minutes.
- Add the shoyu and simmer another 4 to 5 minutes.

Konyaku Preparation
- Place several drops of toasted sesame oil in a cast-iron skillet.
- Add the konyaku bow ties and begin sautéeing.
- Add a dash of schichimi and continue to sautée.
- Add 2 or 3 drops of shoyu and mix with the konyaku.

- Simmer for another 2 to 3 minutes, then remove the konyaku from the pot and place in a small dish.

Mochi Preparation
- Leave this step until right before you are ready to serve the soup!
- Cut the mochi into 1-inch-square pieces.
- Place a small amount of light sesame oil in the bottom of a skillet and turn on the flame.
- Add the mochi and begin frying on a low temperature.
- After 1 to 2 minutes, turn the mochi over and fry on the other side until soft.

To Serve
- Place 3 pieces of konyaku in each bowl.
- Place 1 or 2 pieces of fried mochi in each bowl.
- Garnish with some baby greens.
- Ladle the hot clear soup over top of the ingredients and serve hot.

BEANS

Soaking and Preparing Beans
- Soak beans for 6 to 8 hours or overnight. Discard the soaking water and use fresh water to cook the beans.
- Cook the beans with a 1-inch-long strip of kombu sea vegetable (sometimes labeled as kelp). Kombu makes the beans soft and more digestible.
- Use just enough water to cover the top of the beans. For beans that do not require soaking, such as lentils and split peas, cover the beans with 2 inches of water. Be sure to cook the beans until they are soft before adding any salt. A common mistake is to leave the beans undercooked; undercooked beans are slightly crunchy, not very digestible, and cause gas and bloating.
- Reduce the liquid in the pot before salting the beans. When you add salt, the beans release more liquid. Allow 15 minutes for the salt to blend with the beans.
- When cooking beans on their own, I recommend using a pressure cooker, which drastically reduces cooking time. I prefer boiling my beans when making bean stews.

Cooking Times
- Boiled beans take approximately 3 hours, from start to finish.

- Pressure-cooked beans: timing begins when the beans reach full pressure
- 15 to 20 minutes for quick-cooking varieties, such as black turtle beans, cannellini beans, navy beans, lima beans, black-eyed peas, and pinto beans.
- 50 to 60 minutes for longer-cooking varieties, such as chickpeas, great northern beans, black soybeans, and kidney beans.
- Canned Beans: It is completely acceptable to use canned beans in place of cooking dry beans to save yourself some time. I like using the Eden brand, readily available in many grocery stores. This brand is organic and unseasoned, and the can contains no BPA's.

AZUKI BEANS WITH SEASONAL SWEET VEGETABLES

You may be familiar with the classic version of this dish made with kombu and squash. When squash is not in season, use other seasonal sweet vegetables. Both are delicious, nutritious, and strengthening.

Preparation time: approximately 3 hours
Serves 6 to 8

Ingredients
- 1½ cups azuki beans, washed and soaked 6 to 8 hours. Keep the soaking water and use when cooking the beans.
- 1 medium winter squash such as kabocha, buttercup, or butternut, cut into 2-square-inch pieces. Keep the skin on or leave it off, whatever you prefer.

-or-

- 2 medium onions, diced
- 2 carrots, diced
- 1 to 2 parsnips, diced
- 1 square inch of kombu sea vegetable, rinsed
- Water
- ½ to ¾ teaspoon sea salt
- ¼ to ½ teaspoon shoyu

Preparation

- If you are using onions, cook them on their own for a few minutes before adding the rest of the vegetables and beans. Otherwise, place the kombu and vegetables in the pot.
- Layer the beans on top of the vegetables and add water just to cover the top of the beans.
- Place a lid on the pot, leaving it partially uncovered.
- Bring to a boil, then cover completely. Place a flame deflector under the pot, lower the flame, and simmer 50 minutes to 1 hour.
- Check the liquid level to ensure that the beans are still covered by liquid. Add additional water if needed or use a wooden utensil to immerse the beans in the liquid.
- Replace the cover and continue to simmer on low until the beans are soft, approximately 1½ hours.
- Lightly season with the sea salt and gently fold the ingredients over to blend the salt.
- Continue to simmer for another 10 minutes.
- Add the shoyu and fold to blend. Continue to simmer for another 7 minutes, then serve.

LENTIL SWEET POTATO STEW

This stew is a riff on Azuki Beans with Sweet Vegetables. This is a slightly lighter version, perfect for warmer weather or relaxing your overall condition. This dish is so naturally sweet that it requires very little seasoning.

Preparation time: approximately 3 hours
Serves 6 to 8

Ingredients
- 2 cups green or brown lentils, sorted and washed
- 3 cups sweet potato, peeled and diced
- 2½ cups diced onion
- 1½ cups diced carrot
- Water
- 1-inch strip kelp or kombu
- ¾ teaspoon sea salt

Preparation
- Place the onions in a pot with 2 cups water and bring to a boil.
- Add the kelp, lower the flame, and simmer the onions for 3 to 4 minutes.
- Layer the sweet potato on top of the onions, then add the carrots, then add the lentils.
- Add enough water to cover the lentils by 2 inches.
- Bring the water to a boil. Skim off any excess foam.
- Cover the pot, lower the flame, place a flame deflector under the pot, and simmer for 55 to 60 minutes.
- Remove the cover and check the water level. Add more water to just cover the lentils if necessary. Otherwise, use a wooden spoon to immerse the lentils under the liquid. Re-cover and simmer on low until the lentils are soft, about 1 to 1½ hours.

- Remove the cover and use a wooden utensil to fold the top into the bottom. If the stew is creamy, add the sea salt. If the dish is still a little watery, let simmer uncovered until the liquid is reduced and the lentils are creamy in texture, then add the salt. Fold the top into the bottom to blend all of the ingredients.
- Partially cover the pot and simmer for another 15 to 20 minutes.

CHICKPEA STEW

Preparation time: approximately 2 hours
Serves 4 to 6

Ingredients
- 1 cup chickpeas, washed and soaked
- 1-inch-square piece of kombu
- 2 onions, diced
- 2 stalks celery, sliced thin
- 2 to 3 carrots, diced
- Water
- ½ to ¾ teaspoon sea salt
- ¼ teaspoon shoyu
- Finely chopped fresh herbs, optional

Preparation
- Pour the soaking liquid off of the beans and rinse them several times.
- Place onions in a pressure cooker with a small amount of water to cover, then bring to a boil.

- Add the kombu and allow the onions to cook for another 4–5 minutes.
- Layer the celery on top of the onions, then the carrots, and then the chickpeas.
- Add enough water just to cover the top of the beans.
- Bring to a boil and skim off any foam.
- Place the lid on the pressure cooker and bring to full pressure.
- Place a flame deflector under the pot, lower the flame, and cook for 50 minutes.
- Allow the pressure to come down naturally or run cold water over the bottom of the pot until the pressure releases.
- Remove the lid and test one of the beans to see if it is thoroughly cooked. If the beans are tender, season with sea salt and cook for another 15 to 20 minutes, partially covered. Let any excess liquid cook off before adding the shoyu.
- Add the shoyu and cook for another 5 minutes, then the fresh herbs, if using.

SAVORY LENTIL STEW WITH SAUTÉED ONIONS AND LEEKS

Preparation time: approximately 3 hours
Serves 8

Ingredients
- 3 cups brown or French lentils, sorted and rinsed
- 3 medium onions, diced, approximately 4 cups
- 1-inch piece kombu or kelp
- 6 cups water

- 1 cup thinly sliced leeks
- 2 tablespoons olive oil
- 1¾ teaspoons sea salt, total
- 1¼ teaspoons shoyu
- Splash of white wine
- Red and/or black pepper, optional
- 1 to 2 cloves of garlic, finely chopped, optional
- Finely chopped fresh herbs, such as basil, optional

Preparation
- Place the onions in a pot together with the sea vegetable and 1 cup of water.
- Bring the mixture to a boil and cook for 4 to 5 minutes.
- Add the lentils and enough water to cover by two inches. Bring to a boil and skim off any foam that rises to the top.
- Cover the pot. Place a flame deflector under the pot, lower the flame, and simmer on low for 45 to 50 minutes.
- Lift the lid and check the water level. If most of the water is absorbed, add additional water to cover the top of the lentils. You can also use a wooden spoon to immerse the lentils under the cooking liquid.
- Cover and continue to cook until the beans are soft, approximately 1 to 1½ hours. When the beans are tender, add 1¼ teaspoons sea salt. Fold the top into the bottom to blend the salt throughout the dish.
- In a separate skillet, heat 2 tablespoons of olive oil on a low flame.
- Add the onions and begin sautéeing. When the onions begin to change color add ⅛ teaspoon sea salt, and ¼ cup water, and continue to sautée for 5 minutes.
- Add the leeks and another ¼ cup of water, and sautée for another 5 minutes.
- Add the shoyu and mix with the sautéed vegetables.
- Add the sautéed vegetables to the lentil pot and add the remaining ¼ teaspoon salt.

- Add a splash of white wine and a drizzle of olive oil.
- Gently fold the bottom layer to the top to blend all the seasonings with the lentils. Simmer for another 5 minutes to blend all the ingredients thoroughly, and serve.

HEARTY LENTIL STEW WITH FRIED BREAD

This recipe is a hit with everyone. The fried bread adds a whole other dimension of satisfaction.

Preparation time: approximately 3 hours
Serves 8

Ingredients
- 2 cups lentils, sorted and washed
- 2 medium size onions, diced
- 1 cup diced carrots
- ½ cup diced celery
- 1-inch strip kombu, rinsed
- ½ to ¾ teaspoons sea salt
- Water
- ½ teaspoon shoyu
- Good-quality sake or red wine, optional
- 2 or 3 slices unyeasted sourdough bread
- Safflower oil

Cookware and Utensils
- Heavy pot with lid; I like using a porcelain-coated cast-iron pot for this dish.
- Cast-iron pot for deep-frying
- Wooden spoon
- Wooden chopsticks

Preparation

- Place onions in the heavy pot and add water to just cover the onions. Bring to a gentle boil and add the kombu. Cook for 2 to 3 minutes or until you notice a slight change in the color of the onions.
- Add the remaining ingredients in the following order: celery, carrots, and lentils.
- Add enough water to cover the lentils by 2 inches and bring to a boil.
- Place a lid on the pot, lower the flame, place a flame deflector under the pot, and simmer on low for approximately 45 minutes.
- Check the water level to assure there is enough water for the lentils to continue to cook. If the lentils appear dry, add just enough water to cover. The lentils should be a little juicy before adding the bread, since the bread will absorb a good amount of liquid and thicken the stew.
- If the water level is slightly lower than the lentils, take a wooden spoon and immerse the lentils under the liquid.
- Continue to cook the beans until they are soft, then add the sea salt.
- Gently fold the mixture over to blend the salt, and simmer on low for 15 minutes.
- Season with shoyu, fold again, and simmer for 7 minutes.
- Add the deep-fried bread and simmer another 5 minutes, then add the red wine or sake and simmer another 5 minutes.

Deep-Fried Bread

- Fill the pot with 3 inches of oil and heat to 350 degrees
- Place the bread in the hot oil and fry on each side until golden brown.
- Place fried bread on an unbleached paper towel to drain off excess oil.
- Cut into squares or break into pieces.

WHITE BEANS WITH SAUTÉED ONIONS AND KALE

Preparation time: 15 to 20 minutes
Serves 4

Ingredients
- 1½ to 2 cups pre-cooked white beans
- 2 tablespoons olive oil
- 1½ cups diced onion
- 3 to 4 leaves kale, stems separated from the leaves and sliced thin and leaves chopped. You can also substitute broccoli or escarole for the kale.
- 1 cup water
- ¾ to 1 teaspoon sea salt

Preparation
- Pour the olive oil into a skillet and gently heat on medium-low heat. Add the onions and begin to sautée.
- When the onions are evenly coated with oil, add a small pinch of sea salt. Add a little more water to keep the pan moist and continue to sautée the onions.
- Add the kale stems and cover. Lower the flame and simmer for 2 minutes.
- Add the leaves and the additional water. Cover and simmer for another 2 minutes.
- Add the precooked beans and the sea salt. Gently fold the top into the bottom to blend all of the ingredients together.
- Cover and simmer for 7 minutes.
- Remove the cover, add a drizzle of olive oil, and season to taste with pepper.
- Gently fold to blend the seasoning with the beans and greens.

WHITE BEANS WITH SAUTÉED CABBAGE, ONIONS, AND CARAWAY

My father, Jared Schwalm, came up with this creation.

Preparation time: 15 minutes
Serves 4

Ingredients
- 1 cup onions, diced or cut into ¼-inch half-moons
- 2 cups green head cabbage, sliced thin
- 2 cups cooked white beans
- 2 tablespoons extra virgin olive oil
- ½ to ¾ teaspoon sea salt
- ½ teaspoon umeboshi vinegar
- 1 to 2 tablespoons caraway seeds
- A dash of celery seed, about 1/16 teaspoon

Preparation
- Gently heat 2 tablespoons of olive oil in a cast-iron pot.
- Add the onions and begin to sautée.
- When the onions begin to sweat, add a pinch of sea salt and a little water to the pan. Add the cabbage and continue to sautée.
- Add a sprinkle of caraway and a dash of celery seed.
- Add the white beans, a generous pinch of salt, a dash of pepper, and blend to combine.
- Reduce flame and continue to sautée slowly for another 2–3 minutes.
- Add a dash of umeboshi vinegar at the end of cooking, and mix well.
- Place in a serving dish and cover with a bamboo mat.

ITALIAN-STYLE WHITE BEANS AND GREENS

Preparation time: 10 to 15 minutes
Serves 4 to 5

Ingredients
- 1½ to 2 cups cooked cannellini beans
- 4 cups chopped broccoli rabe, stems separated from the flowers and leaves
- 2 to 3 tablespoons olive oil
- ¾ teaspoon sea salt
- ¾ cup water or bean cooking liquid
- 1 to 2 cloves of garlic, sliced thin or left whole
- Red pepper flakes, to taste

Preparation
- Gently heat 2 tablespoons of olive oil in a cast-iron or sautée pan.
- Add the stems of the greens and begin to sautée.
- Add a little liquid, the garlic, and a good pinch of pepper flakes.
- Add the flowers, the leaves, and a pinch of salt.
- Cover the pot and simmer for a minute.
- Add the beans and the additional salt. Gently fold to blend all the ingredients and simmer for 5 minutes.
- Add a drizzle of olive oil and continue to simmer for another 2 to 3 minutes.

Variation
- Use broccoli or escarole in place of the broccoli rabe.

M' PANATA, OR WHITE BEANS WITH GREENS AND FRIED BREAD

I first tried this recipe at one of our favorite South Philadelphia restaurants, Ristorante Tre Scallini. My version of this recipe is inspired by Chef Francesca DiRenzo's traditional recipe from her hometown, Monteroduni, Isernia in the Molise region of Italy. I think you will find this dish to be one of the most delicious and satisfying bean dishes of all time.

Preparation time: 10 to 15 minutes
Serves 4

Ingredients
- 1½ to 2 cups pre-cooked cannellini beans
- 4 cups chopped broccoli rabe, stems separated from the leaves and the flowers
- 2 to 4 pieces broken bread crumbs, sautéed in olive oil
- ¾ teaspoon sea salt
- 2 to 3 tablespoons extra virgin olive oil
- A dash red pepper flakes
- 1 to 2 cloves of garlic, sliced thin or left whole
- ½ cup water

Preparation
- Gently heat the olive oil in a sautée pan.
- Add the stems and begin to sautée.
- Add a little water and the garlic and pepper flakes.
- Add the flowers, the leaves, and a pinch of salt.
- Cover the pot and simmer for a minute, then add the bread crumbs.
- Add the beans and the remainder of the salt. Gently fold to blend all of the ingredients.
- Simmer for 5 minutes, or until the bread softens.
- Add a drizzle of olive oil and continue to simmer for another 2 to 3 minutes.

- Variation: I have used kale in place of broccoli rabe, also very yummy!

REFRIED BEANS

Preparation time: 15 minutes
Serves 4 to 6

Ingredients
- 4 cups pre-cooked pinto or turtle beans
- 2 medium onions, diced
- 2 tablespoons extra virgin olive oil
- Water and/or bean cooking liquid
- 1½ to 2 teaspoons sea salt
- 1 to 2 scallions, sliced thin
- Chopped cilantro, sliced jalapeño, or cayenne pepper, optional

Preparation
- Heat the olive oil in a deeper skillet or saucepan.
- Add the onions and begin to sautée.
- When the onions begin to sweat, add a pinch of sea salt and 2 or 3 tablespoon of water or bean cooking liquid. If you are using fresh peppers, add them at this time.
- Continue sautéeing until the onions become translucent.
- Add the beans and the rest of the sea salt.
- Fold to blend the seasoning,
- Place a flame deflector under the pot, lower the flame, and simmer for 10 minutes.
- Use the back of a wooden spoon to mash the beans to your desired texture.
- Garnish with chopped cilantro and scallions.

BEAN PRODUCTS

TOFU

MARINATED TOFU

Marinated tofu can be used in sandwiches, wraps, or salads, or in sushi.
Half a block of tofu will make 3 sandwiches or approximately 6 sushi rolls.

Preparation time: 5 to 7 minutes
Marinate time: minimum 3 hours or overnight or longer

Ingredients
- half a block of organic tofu, firm or extra firm
- 1 part umeboshi vinegar (¼ cup umeboshi vinegar)
- 3 to 4 parts water (¾ to 1 cup water). Use more water for a milder flavor.

Preparation
- Rinse the tofu and cut into half-inch-thick slices or strips.
- Place the tofu on a clean cotton towel or paper towel. Place another towel on top and gently press out excess water.
- Place the cut tofu in a flat Pyrex dish.
- Mix the umeboshi vinegar and water in a measuring cup, then pour over the tofu. The tofu should be fully immersed in the liquid. You can place a bamboo mat on top of the tofu to keep it immersed.
- Allow the tofu to marinate at least 3 hours. I like to make this and let it sit overnight.

SIMMERED TOFU

Preparation time: 10 minutes
Half a block of tofu will make 3 sandwiches or 6 sushi rolls

Ingredients
- ½ block organic tofu, extra firm
- 2 teaspoons shoyu
- 2 teaspoons umeboshi vinegar
- ½ teaspoon mirin
- 6 teaspoons water

Preparation
- Rinse the tofu and cut into ½-inch-thick slices.
- Measure the liquid ingredients and pour into a stainless-steel sauce or frying pan.
- Place the tofu in the pan and turn on the flame to medium.
- Bring the liquid to a very gentle boil, lower the flame, and simmer for 2 to 3 minutes on each side.
- Remove the tofu from the pot and place on a plate or dish, and allow it to cool before serving.

TOFU CHEESE

Use tofu cheese in salads, in lightly cooked vegetable dishes, or in pasta.

Preparation time: 5 minutes
½ block tofu makes approximately 2 cups tofu cheese

Ingredients
- ½ block organic tofu, extra firm
- ⅛ cup Mitoku Riyugen Umeboshi Vinegar

Preparation
- Rinse the tofu, then place in a bowl. Use one hand to begin crumbling the tofu while also pouring the umeboshi vinegar into the bowl with the other hand. The texture should remain firm.

Tempeh
- Tempeh is a fermented bean product with a dense consistency and texture. It is a delicious source of protein with a hearty bite and is extremely versatile. Tempeh needs to be boiled in order to make it digestible. Either boil or fry it first for a richer flavor.

Fried Tempeh
- Place about ⅛ to ¼ inch of safflower oil in a cast-iron frying pan. Cut tempeh into desired-size pieces. Fry on each side until the tempeh reaches a golden brown color.
- Place the fried tempeh on unbleached paper to drain off excess oil.
- Next, follow the steps for boiled tempeh.

Boiled Tempeh
- Boil the tempeh in a mixture of 9 parts water to 1 part shoyu, a small piece of kombu, and a few slices of ginger. The tempeh will keep in the cooking liquid for up to 1 week.

Tempeh Reuben
- Lightly reheat tempeh in a pan.
- Place a few slices of boiled tempeh on a steamed sourdough bun and top with caramelized onions, sautéed mushrooms, and sauerkraut.

Other Serving Suggestions
- Cut into cubes and add to light vegetable dishes or salads.
- Cut into strips and use in wraps, fajitas, or nori rolls.

SUBSTANTIAL LONG-COOKED VEGETABLE DISHES

These long-cooked vegetable dishes are considered to be substantial because of their strengthening qualities and their ability to provide us with health benefits for up to 3 days.

NISHIME VEGETABLES

Nishime is a style of cooking that creates a settling energetic effect. Vegetables are cut into medium to large chunks and steamed until they become meltingly soft and tender. In nishime-style cooking, a small piece of kombu seaweed is cooked with the vegetables. The use of kombu, together with the longer cooking time, brings out the protein and carbohydrate qualities in the dish. Nishime is also a layered dish: lighter vegetables are layered on the bottom, followed by round vegetables in the middle, and root vegetables on top. From an energetic perspective, layering this dish enhances its settling qualities. This dynamic cooking method provides us with lasting energy, harmonizes our central organs, and keeps our blood sugar stable.

Preparation time: about 45 minutes
A 1-quart pot yields approximately 4 to 5 servings

Ingredients
- 1-square-inch piece of kombu or kelp sea vegetable, rinsed and/or soaked

327

- $1/16$ to $1/8$ teaspoon sea salt
- $1/8$ to $1/4$ teaspoon shoyu
- Water to cover the bottom of the pot by $1/4$ to $1/2$ inch
- A variety of vegetables cut into 1-to-2-inch chunks. I recommend using sweet vegetables with this dish (refer to vegetable list).
- Round vegetables, cut into wedges or half-rounds.
- Root vegetables, cut using a partial or full roll cut about 1 to 2 inches in length
- Hearty-style leafy greens (such as celery or leeks)
- On occasion you can also use dried shiitake mushrooms in nishime cooking

Cookware
- This dish works best using a heavy pot with a tight-fitting lid. The dish will also turn out much better if the vegetables fit tightly into the pot, leaving very little space. As mentioned above, a 1-quart pot will yield 4–5 servings.

Preparation
- Place kombu on the bottom of the pot.
- Add the first layer of vegetables.
- Add $1/4$ to $1/2$ inch water to cover the bottom of the pot.
- Continue layering the vegetables.
- Add a tiny pinch of sea salt, cover, and bring to a boil over a medium flame. When the water begins to boil, steam will begin to build inside the pot. You may see the steam or notice a little condensation on the side of the pot. You may even hear the water begin to boil. All these signs are an indication that the water inside the pot is boiling.
- Turn the flame down and simmer on low for an average of 25 to 30 minutes, or until the vegetables are tender. The cooking times will vary, depending on the vegetables you use and the size of the pieces.
- Remove the lid and lightly season with a few drops of shoyu.

- Place the lid back on the pot, then pick up the pot and give it a gentle shake to blend the shoyu with any liquid remaining in the pot. Return the pot to the stove and cook for another 4 minutes.
- Remove the pot from the stove and let it stand for a few minutes before placing the vegetables in a serving dish.

ARAME WITH SWEET VEGETABLES

Preparation time: 30 to 40 minutes
Serves 6

Ingredients
- ½ package arame, about 25 grams, soaked until soft, soaking water discarded
- 4 cups onions, sliced into ¼-inch half-moons
- 2½ cups carrots, cut into thin matchsticks
- water, approximately ½ cup
- 1/16 teaspoon sea salt
- ¾ to 1 teaspoon shoyu
- ¼ teaspoon mirin
- ⅛ to ¼ teaspoon sesame oil, optional

Preparation
- Place the onions in a pot with enough water to cover, and turn flame to medium-low.
- When you notice the onions begin to "sweat," add a pinch of sea salt.
- Continue to cook the onions for 3 minutes.

- Layer the carrots on top of the onions and the arame on top of the carrots.
- Add enough water to reach the bottom portion of the arame.
- Cover and bring to a boil on a medium-high flame.
- Reduce the heat to medium-low and simmer for 15 minutes.
- Remove the lid and check the level of the liquid in the pot. There should be about 1½ inches of liquid left in the bottom of the pot. If there is still too much liquid in the pot, crack the lid and allow some of the liquid to reduce before seasoning.
- Add the sesame oil if using, followed by the shoyu.
- Add the mirin.
- Gently fold to blend the seasoning with the ingredients.
- Replace the cover, reduce the heat, and simmer on low for another 5 minutes.

Variations
- For a richer taste, layer crumbled tofu under the arame.
- For a lighter dish, add green peas, snow peas, or edamame at the end of cooking.

ROOTS AND GREENS

Preparation time: 10 to 20 minutes
Serves 3 to 8, depending on the size of the vegetable. One bunch of radishes or turnips will serve 3 to 4, while a daikon radish will serve 6 to 8.

Ingredients
- Choose one of the following: daikon, red radish, turnip, or carrots
- Separate the roots from the stems and leaves, making sure to leave the small connection between the root and stems intact on the root. Cut root portion into matchsticks or half-rounds, or dice them. Finely chop the stems and leaves, separating the leafy parts from the thicker portions of the stems.
- 1/16 teaspoon sea salt
- 1/8 to 1/4 teaspoon shoyu
- 1/4 to 1/2 cup water

Preparation
- Gently heat enough water to cover the bottom of the pan.
- Add the roots and begin sautéeing. If you are using carrots, add 1/2 teaspoon sesame oil to the pan when sautéeing.
- When the roots begin to "sweat," add a tiny pinch of salt and continue to sautée.
- Add about 1/4 cup water, cover, and simmer a few minutes until the roots are about halfway cooked.
- Pull the roots to one side of the pot and add the stems. Fold the roots over the stems, cover, and continue to simmer for 2 to 3 minutes.
- Once again, move the roots and stems to one side, add the leaves, and fold the roots on top of the greens. Allow to simmer another minute before lightly seasoning with the shoyu. Fold the top into the bottom to blend everything together.

CLASSIC KINPIRA

This dish is delicious and hearty. It it is helpful for strengthening blood quality, the bones, and the central nervous system.

Preparation time: 30 to 40 minutes
Serves 6

Ingredients
- 2 cups burdock, cut into thin matchsticks or shaved
- 2 cups carrots, cut into thin matchsticks or shaved slightly thicker than the burdock
- 2 cups lotus root, cut into half-rounds
- ¼ teaspoon light or toasted sesame oil
- 1/16 teaspoon sea salt
- ½ cup water
- Shoyu, approximately ½ teaspoon
- Mirin, approximately ⅛ teaspoon
- Fresh ginger juice, to taste, or shichimi (Japanese Seven Spice)

Preparation
- Add several drops of sesame oil to the skillet and gently heat on a medium-low flame.
- Add the burdock to the pan and begin to sautée.
- When the burdock is coated evenly with oil, add a pinch of sea salt and continue to sautée until the color begins to deepen, approximately 4 minutes.
- Add the lotus root and sautée until it begins to sweat, then add the carrot.
- Add a little water to the bottom of the skillet, then cover and simmer until vegetables are tender, about 7 to 9 minutes.
- Lightly season with the shoyu and mirin, cover, and cook another 4 to 5 minutes.
- At the very end of cooking, add a squeeze of fresh-grated ginger juice or a dash of shichimi.

SWEET VEGETABLE KINPIRA

This is a lighter version of the "classic" sauté and simmer style using sweet vegetables.

Preparation time 30 to 40 minutes
Serves 4

Ingredients
- 2 cups onion, cut into ¼-inch-thick half-moons
- 2 cups root and/or round vegetables, cut into thin matchsticks or slices
- ¼ to ½ teaspoon light sesame oil
- ¹⁄₁₆ to ⅛ teaspoon sea salt
- ½ cup water
- ¼ teaspoon shoyu
- Optional: fresh grated ginger juice

Preparation
- Pour the sesame oil into a skillet, turn on the flame to medium-low to gently heat the oil.
- Add the onions and begin to sautée. When you notice a slight change in color, add a small pinch of sea salt.
- Add approximately ¼ cup water and continue sautéeing until the onions become translucent.
- Add the harder, more fibrous vegetables to the pan and let cook 1 minute. Then add the rest of the vegetables and continue to sautée.
- Add just enough water to keep the pan moist, then cover and simmer until the vegetables are tender.
- Lightly season with a few drops of shoyu.
- Fold to blend the seasoning, cover, and simmer for another 4 to 5 minutes.
- Turn off the flame, then add a squeeze of fresh-grated ginger juice.
- Gently fold to blend with the vegetables.
- Place in a serving dish and cover with a bamboo mat.

CANDIED SWEET POTATOES

Preparation time: 30 minutes
Serves 2, using 1 medium sweet potato per person

Ingredients
- 2 sweet potatoes, peeled and cut lengthwise into 2-inch-thick slices
- 2 tablespoons brown rice syrup
- 1 tablespoon barley malt
- ½ to 1 teaspoon pure maple syrup
- 1 teaspoon extra virgin olive oil
- Water
- Small pinch sea salt, between ¹⁄₁₆ and ⅛ teaspoon

Cookware
- This recipe works best using a wide, cast-iron saucepan with a heavy lid.

Preparation
- Place the sweet potatoes in the pan with just enough water to cover the bottom of the pan. Cover and bring to a boil.
- Lower the flame and steam on low heat for 5 minutes.
- Remove the lid and drizzle a little olive oil over the sweet potatoes, then add a pinch of salt, cover, and continue to steam for 10 minutes.
- In a separate bowl, mix the rice syrup, barley malt, and maple syrup together. Pour over top of the sweet potatoes, replace lid, and continue to cook until the potatoes are tender. As the potatoes cook, the sauce will reduce, forming a sweet glaze.

MEDITERRANEAN SAUTÉED VEGETABLES

This is one of my "go-to" dishes when I want something quick with a little more substance. It is simple to prepare, yet offers a nourishing and satisfying quality. As an added bonus, everyone who tries it seems to love it!

Preparation time: 10 to 15 minutes
Serves 4 to 6

Ingredients
- 1 bunch of broccoli or a small head of cauliflower, or round green cabbage
- ⅛ to ¼ teaspoon sea salt
- 2 to 3 tablespoons extra virgin olive oil
- ¼ to ½ cup of water

Cookware
- Deep stainless-steel or cast-iron sautée pan with lid

Preparation
- Cut vegetables into medium to larger florets, or into 2-inch pieces if using cabbage.
- Peel and slice the stems into matchsticks proportionate to the size of the florets.
- Add enough water to cover the bottom of the pan, then turn on the flame to medium-low.
- Place the stems and florets in the pan, cover, turn the flame to medium, and steam for 2 minutes.
- Remove the lid and drizzle olive oil over the vegetables, then add a pinch of sea salt.
- Cover and continue to steam for another minute.
- Remove the lid and gently fold to blend the seasonings.
- Return the cover and continue cooking about 7 minutes, or until the vegetables reach the desired texture. The longer

you cook the vegetables, the sweeter they will be. Remove vegetables from the pot, place in a serving dish, and cover with a bamboo mat.

SAUTÉED BROCCOLI RABE

Preparation time: 7 to 10 minutes
Serves 2

Ingredients
- 1 bunch broccoli rabe, stems, leaves, and florets separated.
- 2 to 3 tablespoons extra virgin olive oil
- ⅛ to ¼ teaspoon sea salt
- Water
- Optional: dried red pepper flakes

Preparation
- Cut the stems on an angle into 2-inch-long pieces.
- Add enough water to cover the bottom of the pan, then turn the flame to medium-low and place the stems in the pan.
- Cover and steam for 1 to 2 minutes.
- Add the leaves, cover, and steam for another minute.
- Add the florets, a drizzle of olive oil, and a pinch of salt.
- Gently fold the ingredients to blend the seasoning and continue to sautée until tender but still slightly crunchy.
- Place in a serving bowl and cover with a bamboo mat.

LIGHT VEGETABLE DISHES

Lightly cooked vegetable dishes are important to include with every meal. They provide us with fresh, uplifting energy and keep our internal condition hydrated. When we eat lightly cooked vegetable dishes on a regular basis, we do not need to drink gallons of water every day. Because these dishes are cooked quickly, they sharpen our reflexes, allowing us to think and react more quickly, a wonderful benefit for both work and play!

QUICK STEAMED GREENS

Quick steamed greens are a lightly cooked vegetable dish with more settling energetic qualities. Steamed greens should be bright, crunchy, and a little deeper in color than blanched greens. Use only one type of leafy green per serving. Broccoli can be considered a leafy green.

2 to 3 leaves serves 1 person
Preparation time: 1 to 2 minutes

Ingredients
- Choose a leafy green from the "regular use" list.

Cookware

- A stainless-steel pot and a steamer basket. I prefer the type of basket that sits on top of the pot made from bamboo or stainless steel over the collapsible steamer baskets that fit inside the pot.

Preparation

- Wash the vegetables well to remove unwanted debris and dirt.
- Separate the leaves from the stems with a sharp knife.
- Cut the stems on an angle.
- More fibrous stems should be sliced thinly, approximately ⅛ to ¼ inch in width. Juicier stems (such as bok choy or napa cabbage) may be cut thicker, approximately ½ to 1 inch in length.
- Cut the leaves on an angle, approximately 1 to 2 inches in length.
- Place ¾ to 1 inch of water in the bottom of a pot and place the steamer basket over the pot.
- Cover and turn the flame to medium-high.
- When the pot is filled with steam, add the stems to the basket.
- Cover and steam for 20 seconds or longer. The more fibrous the stem, the longer you will need to cook them, up to 1 minute in some cases.
- Add the leaves, cover and continue steaming for another 30 seconds or longer. Again, the texture of the greens varies according to the vegetable type, the growing season, and the environment.
- When done, the greens should still be crunchy, but tender enough to chew easily.
- Remove the greens from the basket and place in a serving dish. Cover with a sushi mat until serving.
- Optional: For an even lighter, more refreshing effect, add a squeeze of fresh lemon on your greens.

BLANCHED VEGETABLE SALAD

This light and colorful dish is a combination of root, round, and leafy green vegetables. The method of preparation and the combination of the different types of vegetables creates a dynamic energetic effect that helps to activate circulation from deep inside our bodies.

Preparation time: 10 to 15 minutes
Serves 2 to 3

Ingredients
- Choose a minimum of 2 different vegetables, from different categories, or use the combination listed below:
- 4 to 5 leafy greens, thinly sliced 1 inch wide by 2 inches in length
- 1 to 2 cups round vegetables, quartered and sliced thinly
- ½ cup root vegetables, cut into matchsticks ideally not thicker than ½ inch.
- A small pinch of sea salt
- Enough water to fill the pot halfway up

Cookware and Utensils
- A stainless-steel pot
- A "spider" or mesh vegetable skimmer (to remove vegetables from the water)
- Several plates
- Bamboo mats

Preparation
- Fill a pot halfway with water and bring the water to a boil over a medium flame.
- Add a pinch of sea salt.
- In an open pot, blanch one vegetable at a time, starting with the mildest in taste and lightest in color. When you add the vegetables, the water may stop boiling.

- When the color of the vegetables brightens, remove the vegetable from the pot and place on a plate. Cover with a sushi mat and drain off any excess water.
- After the water returns to a boil, add the next vegetable and repeat the process.
- Repeat the entire process for all of the vegetables.
- Allow the vegetables to cool, then gently mix in a bowl.
- Cover with a sushi mat until ready to serve.
- Optional: Sprinkle brown rice vinegar or umeboshi vinegar on your blanched salad.

QUICK SAUTÉED VEGETABLES—RED ONION, BOK CHOY, CARROT

Preparation time: 10 to 15 minutes
Serves 4

Ingredients
- 1 medium onion, sliced in thin half-moons
- 1½ cups root vegetables, cut into thin matchsticks
- 4 to 6 leafy greens leaves, stems and leaves separated and cut ½ inch thick on the angle
- 1 to 2 teaspoons light sesame oil or 1 tablespoon extra virgin olive oil
- ⅛ teaspoon sea salt
- ¼ to ½ cup water
- Several drops shoyu

Note: Sautéed vegetables cook quickly. They should be bright, colorful, and crunchy.

Preparation
- Gently heat the oil in a saucepan, skillet, or other sautée pan.
- Tilt the pan so the oil spreads out evenly and lightly coats the bottom.
- Add the onions, turn up the flame, and begin to sautée.
- Add a little water, a pinch of sea salt, and continue to sautée for 2 minutes.
- Add the leafy green stems and more water if needed to keep the pan moist, continue to sautée.
- Add the leaves, followed by the root vegetables, and continue sautéeing.
- When the colors begin to deepen, approximately 1 to 2 minutes, you are ready to season. Make sure you have a little juice in the bottom of the pan. If the pan is dry, add a little more water.
- Add a few drops of shoyu to the juice, then continue sautéeing to blend the seasoning.
- Remove the vegetables from the skillet, place in a serving dish, and cover with a sushi mat until ready to serve.
- Optional: Add a little spice, such as red pepper flakes or ginger juice. Chili pepper may be added after the onions at the beginning of cooking. A squeeze of fresh ginger juice may be added at the very end of cooking.

QUICK SAUTÉED LEAFY GREENS

This is a light preparation style where I begin by slightly steaming the greens, then adding oil and seasoning. The greens are juicy but still retain their crunchy texture.

Preparation time: 7 to 8 minutes
Serves 2 to 4

Ingredients
- ½ to 1 bunch leafy greens, washed and cut into larger pieces (approximately 2 to 3 inches in length and width). Baby greens may be kept whole.
- ⅛ teaspoon sea salt
- 1 tablespoon extra virgin olive oil or several drops of light sesame oil.
- If using olive oil, season only with sea salt.
- Season with 5 to 6 drops of shoyu if using sesame oil.

Preparation
- Gently heat just enough water to cover the bottom of the pan.
- Add the stems, cover, and steam for 20 to 30 seconds.
- Add the leaves, cover, and steam for another 10 seconds.
- Drizzle a little oil over the top, then add a little sea salt and fold to blend the seasoning.
- Finish cooking the greens using a sautée method, approximately 20 to 30 more seconds. Place in a serving dish and cover with a sushi mat.
- Optional: add fresh garlic, red pepper flakes, or fresh ginger juice.

ASIAN-STYLE MUSTARD GREENS

Preparation time: 5 to 7 minutes
Serves 2 to 3

Ingredients
- ½ bunch washed mustard greens, stems and leaves separated
- 2 or 3 drops toasted sesame oil
- 5 or 6 drops shoyu
- 3 drops mirin
- Water

Preparation
- Place a small amount of water in a skillet (enough just to cover the bottom of the pan) and turn on the flame.
- Add the stems, cover, and steam for 30 seconds to 1 minute.
- Remove the lid, add the leaves, cover, and steam for an additional 20 to 30 seconds.
- Remove the lid, and then add 2–3 drops of toasted sesame oil, 5 drops of shoyu, and 2–3 drops of mirin.
- Mix all ingredients together in the pan, using a wooden spatula or chopsticks.
- Place in a serving dish and cover with a sushi mat.

Variations
- Use spicy toasted sesame oil, cayenne pepper, or shichimi.
- Use watercress, baby kale, or dandelion in place of mustard greens.

SALADS

Raw salads refresh and relax our condition. There are many varieties of lettuces and leafy greens that taste great in salads. Even though it is not usually thought of as a "healthy" choice, I love using iceberg lettuce because it is so refreshing, due to its high moisture content. You can also mix and match the greens you use in your salads.

SIMPLE ICEBERG SALAD

Preparation time: 10 minutes
Serve 2 to 4

Ingredients
- ½ head iceberg lettuce
- 1 medium cucumber, cut into ½-inch-thick (or thinner) slices

Optional:
- Grated carrots or feathery thin matchsticks
- 1 to 2 red radishes, sliced into thin half-rounds
- Tofu cheese: ⅓ block tofu, crumbled and seasoned with ⅛ cup umeboshi vinegar

Preparation
- Remove the outer leaves and center core of the lettuce.
- Break open the head of lettuce and wash.
- Drain off the excess water. Use a salad spinner or clean cotton dish towels to absorb the excess moisture.
- Break the lettuce up into a bowl.
- Add any additional vegetables you desire and/or tofu cheese.
- Toss together and serve with your favorite dressing.

Dressings:
- A few drops of umeboshi vinegar
- A few drops of brown rice vinegar
- A squeeze of fresh lemon or tangerine
- A few drops of balsamic or red wine vinegar

ARUGULA SALAD

Preparation time: 10 minutes
Serves 2 to 4

Ingredients
- 5 ounces arugula, washed
- Tofu cheese: ⅓ block tofu, crumbled and seasoned with ⅛ cup umeboshi vinegar
- ⅓ cup lightly toasted pine nuts
- ½ to 1 tablespoon olive oil
- Pinch sea salt, about 1/16 teaspoon
- Umeboshi vinegar
- Fresh-squeezed lemon juice to taste
- Fresh-cracked black pepper, if desired

Preparation
- Place arugula in a bowl and add a drizzle of olive oil and a tiny pinch of sea salt, then toss to blend.
- Add the tofu cheese and lemon, and toss to blend.
- Place in a serving dish, and garnish with toasted pine nuts.

Variations
- Add some thin slices of fresh pear or apple.
- Add thin slices of cooked beets.

ARUGULA SALAD WITH SAUTÉED MUSHROOMS

Preparation time: 10 minutes
Serves 4

Ingredients
- 5 ounces arugula, washed
- ½ to 1 pound fresh mushrooms, such as oyster, beech, or maitake
- ½ red onion, sliced into half-moons
- Tofu cheese (see above)
- Olive oil
- Pinch sea salt, about ¹⁄₁₆ teaspoon
- ¼ teaspoon shoyu
- 3 or 4 drops mirin

Preparation
- Place the washed arugula in a bowl, and add the tofu cheese on top of the arugula.

Mushrooms

- Heat 1 to 2 tablespoons of olive oil in a pan.
- Add the red onion and begin to sautée.
- Add a little water, a pinch of sea salt, and 2 or 3 drops of umeboshi vinegar.
- Add the beech mushrooms, cover the pot, and simmer for 1 minute.
- Add the oyster mushrooms and continue to sautée.
- Add the maitake mushrooms and lightly season with the shoyu and mirin.
- Sautée for another minute to cook the mushrooms and blend the seasonings together.
- Pour the sautéed mushrooms over the arugula and tofu cheese.
- Lightly toss all ingredients together and serve.

VEGAN AVOCADO CAESAR SALAD
WITH TEMPEH CROUTONS

Preparation time: 30 to 40 minutes, including the time to cook the tempeh
Serves 4 to 6

Ingredients

- 1 head romaine hearts, washed
- 1 package of tempeh, cooked and cut into inch cubes (see tempeh recipe in the bean section)
- 1 small red onion, cut into ⅛-inch-thick half-moons

- Guacamole or avocado slices (½ to 1 avocado)

Preparation
- Slice the red onion and place in a bowl. Add 1/16 teaspoon of sea salt and 2 or 3 drops of umeboshi vinegar. Very gently rub the salt and vinegar into the onion until you see the color deepen. Set aside until you are ready to assemble your salad.
- Wash the romaine and remove any excess water using a salad spinner or cotton towel.
- Break the lettuce into a bowl.
- Add the red onion and the tempeh and lightly toss with your hands or wooden utensils.
- Add a little freshly made guacamole, toss to coat the lettuce. If you do not have time to make guacamole, add some fresh avocado slices.
- Drizzle a little umeboshi vinegar over the entire salad, then toss to blend the ingredients.

SUSAN'S GUACAMOLE

Preparation time: 15 to 20 minutes
Serves 2 to 4

Ingredients
- 1 avocado
- ½ cup finely diced onion
- Freshly sliced jalapeño pepper, center vein and seeds removed (optional)
- ¼ cup finely chopped cilantro

- Fresh lime juice, to taste
- 1½ to 1¾ teaspoons umeboshi vinegar

Preparation
- Dice the onion and place in a pyrex bowl. Add ⅟₁₆ teaspoon sea salt to the onion and gently mix. Add ½ teaspoon umeboshi vinegar to the onions, mix all ingredients together with your hands, and set aside while you prepare the other ingredients.
- Cut the avocado in half and remove the pit and the rind.
- Place avocado in a bowl together with the marinated onions and the liquid from the onions. Add the cilantro and peppers and the remaining ¾ to 1 teaspoon umeboshi vinegar to taste. Add the lime juice and gently mix.

This recipe keeps longer than other guacamole recipes because of the umeboshi vinegar. The pickled onions balance the rich vegetable fat of the avocado. You can store the guacamole in a glass or earthenware bowl together with the pit (to maintain freshness). Remove the pit before serving. Serve with good-quality corn chips (again made with non-GMO, organic corn and sea salt), lightly blanched or raw carrots or celery sticks, or top off a vegan rice and bean burrito.

PICKLES

Pickles are an important part of creating healthy digestion. Ideally you should try to include a small 1-or-2-tablespoon serving of pickles almost daily. Because pickles are salty, it is important to stick to just one small serving. We recommend having pickles with meals about five times per week.

You can purchase naturally fermented pickles at the local health-food shop or at the farmers' market. When shopping for pickles, such as sauerkraut, look for organic ingredients and sea salt. There should be no preservatives listed on the label.

You can also try making your own pickles at home. It's quite easy, and you can control what vegetables and how much salt go into your homemade pickles. Homemade pickles are also delicious!

QUICK UMEBOSHI VINEGAR PICKLES

Preparation time: 15 minutes
Minimum fermentation time: 3 hours
Serving size is approximately 2 tablespoons

Ingredients
- Choose one vegetable or a combination of vegetables. Here are some of my favorites:
- Daikon radish or red radish, sliced into half-rounds on the angle

- Cauliflower florets
- Turnips, sliced into thin half-rounds
- Red onion, sliced into ¼-to-½-inch-thick half-moons
- Lotus root, cut into half-rounds
- Red or green cabbage, cut into 1-inch squares or thin slices
- 3 to 3½ parts water per 1 part vegetable
- 1 part Mitoku Riyugen Umeboshi Vinegar per 1 part vegetable

Cookware
- Deep pyrex bowl or glass jar
- Small plate or dish
- Sushi mat or cheesecloth

Preparation
- Cut the vegetables and place them in the deep Pyrex bowl.
- Use a liquid measuring cup to measure the liquid ingredients.
- Pour enough liquid to cover the vegetables. Place the small bowl or dish over the vegetables to keep them submerged under the brine.
- Cover the bowl with a sushi mat or cheesecloth and place in a cool, dark area to ferment.
- The thicker-cut vegetables and the heartier vegetables (such as the turnips) will need to be fermented longer than thinly sliced or softer vegetables. I usually let my pickles ferment overnight.
- Umeboshi pickles will keep in the fridge for up to one week.

QUICK CUCUMBER PICKLES

Preparation time: 10 minutes
Fermentation time: 3 hours
Serving size is approximately 1 to 2 tablespoons

Ingredients
- 1 to 2 cucumbers, washed, cut in half lengthwise, seeds removed
- 1 part umeboshi vinegar
- 4 parts water

Preparation
- Slice the cucumber on the angle in ½-inch to 1-inch-thick slices.
- Place the cucumber slices in a bowl.
- Use a liquid measuring cup to measure the liquid ingredients and pour liquid over the cucumbers to cover.
- Cover the bowl with a sushi mat or cheesecloth and place in a cool, dark area to ferment for 3 hours.
- Use within 24 hours so that the pickles stay crispy and fresh.

QUICK PRESSED CUCUMBER AND RED ONION FOR SALADS

Preparation time: 30 minutes

Ingredients
- ½ cucumber, seeds removed and sliced thinly on the angle

- ½ red onion, sliced into ¼ inch-thick half-moons
- ¹⁄₁₆ teaspoon sea salt
- ¼ teaspoon umeboshi vinegar

Preparation
- Place the sliced onion in a prep bowl.
- Add a small pinch of sea salt and use your hands to mix the salt with the onions. Massage the onions for 2 minutes.
- Add the cucumber to the bowl, then continue to massage the vegetables for another 2 to 3 minutes.
- Add the umeboshi vinegar, then use your hands to gently blend the seasonings.
- Cover with a sushi mat and allow the vegetables to sit while you assemble the rest of your salad.
- Add the pressed vegetables to your favorite salad base and enjoy.

DESSERTS

APPLE GRAPE KANTEN DESSERT

Fresh fruit kanten is a clean, refreshing dessert that is the perfect ending to a big meal.

> Preparation time: 20 minutes to make, and approximately 1 hour to set
> Serves 3 to 4

Ingredients
- 2 cups apple juice
- 1 to 2 cups spring or filtered water
- 1 tablespoon agar-agar (also called kanten flakes) per cup of liquid. For three cups of total liquid (apple juice and water), use 3 tablespoons agar-agar.
- 1½ to 2 cups fresh grapes, cut in half and seeds removed

Preparation
- Place the apple juice and water in a pot.
- Add the agar-agar and bring to a slight boil on a medium flame.
- Lower flame and simmer until the kanten dissolves.

- Place the grapes in the serving dish of choice. Use either a large serving dish or individual ramekins. Pour the hot liquid over the fruit and allow the kanten to set, either at room temperature or in the refrigerator.

Variations
- Try using different fruit juices such as grape, white grape, peach, berry, and pear juice. Use different fruit combinations. I like fresh tangerines or cherries.

Serving Suggestions
- Make your kanten look extra-special by using champagne flutes or crystal and garnishing with fresh mint leaves. You can also top your kanten with almond creme or mousse, by blending a little kanten and amasake together.

POACHED PEARS

Preparation time: 15 minutes
Serves 2 to 4

Ingredients
- 2 pears, washed, cored, and quartered
- Water
- $\frac{1}{16}$ teaspoon sea salt
- 1 to 2 tablespoons barley malt
- lemon wedge or balsamic vinegar

Preparation
- Place a small amount of water in a deep sautée pan, just enough to cover the bottom.

- Place pears in the pan and add a tiny pinch of sea salt, cover, and bring to a boil on a medium flame.
- Lower the flame and steam for 5 minutes, then drizzle 1 tablespoon of barley malt over top. Note that the cooking time will vary according to the ripeness, variety, and texture of the pear. The pear should still be slightly crunchy when you add the barley malt.
- Replace the cover and give the pot a gentle shake to mix the sweetener with the cooking liquid.
- Cook pears until they reach the desired texture.
- Squeeze a little fresh lemon or add a little aged balsamic vinegar over top of the pears and gently fold to blend the flavors.
- When the pears reach a desired texture, place in a serving dish. Continue heating the remaining sweet mixture to allow it to reduce, then pour over the plated pears.
- Place in a serving dish.

PANNA COTTA WITH FRESH FRUIT SAUCE

Preparation time: 1½ hours
Serves 4 to 5

Ingredients
- 2 cups amasake
- 1 cup organic non-GMO soy milk or almond milk
- 2 teaspoons agar-agar flakes (also called kanten flakes)
- 1 to 3 teaspoons maple syrup or 1 tablespoon rice syrup
- ½ teaspoon vanilla extract

Preparation

- Pour liquid ingredients into a pot and gently begin to heat on a low flame.
- Add the kanten flakes and bring the liquid to a very gentle boil.
- Lower the flame and simmer until all of the agar-agar is completely dissolved.
- Turn off the flame.
- Add the maple syrup and stir with a wooden spoon to mix well.
- Add the vanilla and stir.
- Pour the liquid into a bowl or mold and allow it to cool.
- When your dessert sets, gently remove it from the mold and place it on a serving dish together with the sauce.

Fresh Fruit Sauce

Ingredients

- Apple or grape juice to cover the bottom of the pan, about ⅛ cup
- 1 cup fresh berries
- Maple syrup or rice syrup, to taste

Preparation

- Add the apple or grape juice to a saucepan with some fresh berries and a few grains of sea salt. Turn on the flame and simmer on low. The liquid will begin to reduce and thicken into a sauce as the berries begin to cook. When the sauce reaches the desired consistency turn off the flame. If the berries are a little tart, you may want to add a little maple syrup or rice syrup to make the sauce sweeter. To serve, place some sauce on a dish, then place the panna cotta on top of the sauce. Garnish with a few fresh berries and a nice fresh sprig of mint.

CARAMEL RICE PUDDING

Preparation time: approximately 1 hour
Serves 2 to 4

Ingredients
- 1 cup organic carnaroli risotto rice
- 5 cups water
- 1 cup apple juice
- ⅛ teaspoon sea salt
- ¼ to ½ teaspoon organic olive oil
- 1 teaspoon vanilla extract
- 2 teaspoons fresh-squeezed orange juice

Cookware and Utensils
- 1 medium stainless-steel pot
- Le Creuset pot or a pot with a heavy bottom
- Wooden spoon for stirring
- Wooden ladle

Preparation
- Heat the apple juice and water together in a pot.
- In a separate, heavier pot, warm the olive oil over a low flame. Add the risotto rice and sautée for 1 to 2 minutes.
- Ladle the warm liquid over the rice, then add the sea salt and stir. Allow the liquid to begin to absorb into the rice almost completely before adding any additional liquid.
- Continue to ladle the liquid into the rice and fold rice after each ladle of liquid is added. When you reach the desired consistency and texture, turn off the flame. If you want a creamier texture, use the entire amount of liquid. If you like the rice to have more texture, use less liquid.
- Add the fresh orange juice and blend with the rice.

Caramel topping
- ½ cup brown rice syrup
- ½ cup barley malt
- 1 tablespoon water
- 2 to 3 drops umeboshi vinegar
- 1 teaspoon fresh-squeezed orange juice

Preparation
- Put the water, rice syrup, and barley malt in a saucepan.
- Add the umeboshi vinegar and mix well with a wooden spoon.
- Gently heat the mixture until it begins to boil around the edges of the pan.
- Turn the flame off. Add the fresh orange juice and mix well.

Serving Suggestions
- Use individual serving dishes. Ladle a little sauce on the bottom, followed by the rice.
- Pour additional sauce on top, and garnish with roasted pecans and fresh berries.
- You can also create a parfait by layering fresh berries between layers of pudding.

AMASAKE ALMOND KANTEN

Preparation time: 30 to 40 minutes to cook and approximately 1 hour to set
Serves 4 to 6

Ingredients
- 2 cups amasake

- 1 cup organic apple juice or cider
- 1 cup water
- 1 to 2 tablespoons barley malt
- 7 teaspoons agar-agar flakes (also known as kanten flakes)
- ½ cup toasted almonds, finely chopped or crushed

Preparation
- Pour all the liquid ingredients in a saucepan and begin to heat over a medium flame.
- As the liquid begins to warm, add the kanten flakes, then bring to a gentle boil.
- Lower the flame and continue to simmer until the agar dissolves completely.
- Add the barley malt and mix well.
- Ladle the liquid into individual serving dishes or into a flat pyrex pan.
- Allow the liquid to cool for a few minutes, then top with the almonds.
- The kanten will begin to set as it cools. You may also allow it to cool in the refrigerator.

PUMPKIN CUSTARD

Preparation time: 1 to 2 hours
Serves 6

Ingredients
- 3¾ cups cooked pumpkin (two 15-ounce cans)
- 1½ cups water

- 1 to 1¼ cups brown rice syrup
- 1 teaspoon maple syrup
- 9 to 10 teaspoons agar-agar (kanten flakes)
- Optional: cinnamon and nutmeg to taste and/or my Grand-
  mother's secret ingredient, a splash of good whiskey!

Preparation
- Mix the cooked pumpkin and water together and place in
  a pot.
- Begin to gently heat the mixture over a low flame.
- Add the kanten flakes and gently cook until the flakes are
  completely dissolved.
- Add rice syrup and stir to blend thoroughly with the pumpkin.

Serving ideas
- Garnish with chopped and toasted pecans and/or almond
  creme. Pumpkin custard also makes a great topping for
  couscous or teff cake, or a filling for pumpkin pie.

STEAMED SEASONAL FRUITS
WITH SWEET KUZU SAUCE

Preparation time: 15 minutes
1 piece of fruit yields 1 to 2 servings

Ingredients
- Fresh peaches, apples, or pears, washed and cored and
  cut into quarters, about 2 to 3 pieces of fruit

- 1 to 2 tablespoons rice syrup
- A pinch of sea salt, about 1/16 teaspoon
- 1 slightly rounded teaspoon kuzu per 1 cup liquid
- 1/2 to 1 teaspoon fresh lemon juice
- Water

Preparation

- Fill a deep, wide skillet with about 1/2 inch to 1 inch of water. Use more water for harder fruits such as apples or pears and less water for softer fruits like peaches. Place fruit in the pot, cut side down.
- Add a tiny pinch of sea salt, turn on the flame to a medium setting, and cover.
- Bring the water to a boil, then lower the flame and gently steam the fruit to the desired texture. The type of fruit you use and the firmness you desire will determine the cooking time. You want the fruit to be tender enough to cut it easily with a spoon but not mushy. Harder fruits take approximately 2 to 5 minutes or longer to cook. Softer fruits may take only 2 to 3 minutes to cook. Check the texture while the fruit is cooking.
- When the fruit Is almost tender, add the rice syrup and cook uncovered for another minute.
- Turn off the flame, remove the fruit from the pan and place it in a serving dish.
- Leave the juice in the pan to make the sauce.
- Measure the kuzu in a separate Pyrex bowl.
- Add 1/4 to 1/3 cup water and dissolve the kuzu, using your fingers to break up any clumps.
- Turn the flame on low and add the dissolved kuzu to the juice in the pan while stirring constantly.
- Continue to stir until the liquid comes to a boil and thickens. Turn off the flame and allow the sauce to sit for a minute.
- Drizzle sauce over the fruits and garnish with fresh mint sprig or shiso leaves, lightly toasted walnuts, or pecans.

BAKED APPLES

Preparation time: 1½ hours
Serves 6 to 8

Ingredients
- 4 apples, washed and cored
- ¼ cup barley malt
- ½ cup rice syrup
- ¼ cup maple syrup
- ¼ teaspoon umeboshi vinegar
- ¼ teaspoon vanilla extract
- 1 cup chopped walnuts
- ½ to 1 cup raisins
- 1 teaspoon extra virgin olive oil
- 1 teaspoon walnut oil
- ⅓ cup apple juice

Cookware
- Deep baking dish
- 2 prep bowls
- Spatula
- Dry and wet measuring cups

Preparation
- Preheat oven to 375 degrees.
- Measure the dry ingredients into a bowl and mix well.
- Measure the wet ingredients and pour into a separate bowl and mix well.
- Make a well in the middle of the dry ingredients, then pour the wet ingredients into the well and mix.
- Pour a tablespoon of olive oil and walnut oil into a dish and mix the oils.
- Dip your hands into the oil, then rub each apple with oil.

- Use the remaining oil to oil the baking pan.
- Pour the apple juice into the bottom of the pan and place the apples in the pan, stem side facing up.
- Fill each core with the sweet nut mixture.
- Bake uncovered for 1 hour or until soft.

STRAWBERRY-BLUEBERRY FRUIT CRUMBLE

This recipe uses strawberries and blueberries, but you can substitute 9 cups of other berries or fruits of your choice.

Preparation time: 1½ hours
Serves approximately 12 to 14

Ingredients

For the fruit filling:
- 4½ cups fresh blueberries, washed and stems removed
- 4½ cups fresh strawberries, washed, stems removed, and quartered
- 6 tablespoons unbleached white flour
- ⅛ to ¼ cup apple juice
- 2 tablespoons rice syrup

For the topping:
- 1 cup whole-wheat pastry flour
- 1 cup cornmeal flour
- 1 cup rolled oats
- ½ cup oat bran flour (or rolled oats whizzed in the blender or food processor)
- ½ cup white flour

- ½ teaspoon sea salt
- ¼ cup barley malt
- ½ cup rice syrup
- ¼ cup maple syrup
- ⅓ cup walnut oil
- ⅓ cup extra virgin olive oil (if possible, choose an olive oil with a buttery finish)
- 1 teaspoon vanilla extract

Preparation
- Preheat oven to 375 degrees.
- Place washed and cut berries in a prep bowl and set aside.
- Use a dry measuring cup to measure the dry topping ingredients into a large prep bowl, and use a pastry blender or two forks to combine well.
- Place the dry topping bowl in the refrigerator while you are preparing the wet ingredients. Measure the wet ingredients into a prep bowl and blend with a spatula.
- Sprinkle the 6 tablespoons of unbleached white flour over the top of the berries. Blend the apple juice and rice syrup together, pour over the fruit, and mix to coat the fruit evenly.
- Oil the baking dish with about 1 teaspoon of olive oil or walnut oil, and add the berry mixture to the dish.
- Take the dry ingredients out of the refrigerator.
- Make a well in the middle of the dry ingredients and add the wet ingredients.
- Blend the wet and dry ingredients together with a pastry blender or two forks. The mixture should form a thick batter.
- Use a spatula to spread the mixture evenly on top of the fruit. Try not to touch the batter with your hands, as the heat and moisture in your hands will affect the texture of the crumble topping.
- Bake uncovered for 30 to 35 minutes.

BROWN RICE CRISPY TREATS

Although these are more of a kids' snack, everyone seems to love eating these sweet, crunchy treats. This quick snack will keep in a tin or glass container for 1 week.

Preparation time: 15 to 20 minutes
Serves 10

Ingredients
- ½ cup barley malt
- ¾ cup maple syrup
- 1 cup organic currants or raisins
- 1 cup organic peanut butter
- 5 cups organic crispy brown rice cereal

Preparation
- Mix barley malt, maple syrup, and peanut butter in a stainless-steel pot. Gently heat on a low flame, then add the fruits and continue to mix. When bubbles appear around the edge of the pot, turn off the flame and add the crispy brown rice cereal. Mix well to blend all the ingredients. Place on an oiled tray to cool a bit, then roll into balls and serve.

Variations
- Substitute almond butter or tahini for the peanut butter. When using tahini, increase the amount of rice cereal by ¼ to ½ cup to maintain a pliable consistency. You can also add grain-sweetened chocolate chips for an extra-special treat.

JUICES

With their light freshness and sweet taste, fresh vegetable and fruit combination juices are perfect for satisfying a sweet craving. They are particularly beneficial to the liver, gallbladder, and pancreas. I like to include juices as a snack or as part of a meal when I create menus for my clients.

Juicers: I like using a slow juicer model for vegetables and hard fruits, as they yield more juice than high-speed juicers do. A hand juicer works well for citrus.

*All vegetable or vegetable-fruit juices are best when they are made fresh; try to consume them immediately after juicing. Here are some of my favorite combinations.

FRESH CARROT JUICE

Preparation time: 5 to 7 minutes
Serves 1

Ingredients
- 4 to 4½ large carrots, or enough to yield one 8-ounce serving of juice

Preparation
- Wash the carrots and cut into 1-inch pieces.
- Place the carrots in a juicer and juice according to your juicer manufacturer's instructions.
- Pour juice into a glass and enjoy immediately.

CARROT-APPLE JUICE

Preparation time: 10 minutes
Serves 2

Ingredients
- 4 large carrots or 1 cup fresh carrot juice
- 2 apples or 1 cup fresh apple juice
- A squeeze of fresh lemon, optional

Preparation
- Wash the carrots and cut into 1-inch-long pieces.
- Wash and core the apple, then cut into 1-inch pieces. Fill a dish with water and a few grains of sea salt and add the sliced apple to prevent it from oxidizing while preparing the juice.
- Place the carrots in a juicer and juice according to your juicer manufacturer's instructions, then do the same with the apple.
- If you are adding the fresh lemon, squeeze it directly into the juice and blend thoroughly with a wooden utensil.
- Pour juice into two glasses and enjoy immediately.

CARROT-APPLE-ORANGE JUICE WITH A TWIST

Preparation time: 10 to 15 minutes
Serves 2

Ingredients
- 4 large carrots or 1 cup fresh carrot juice
- 1 apple or ½ cup fresh apple juice
- 1 large orange, or ½ cup orange juice
- 2 or 3 lemon wedges, sliced 1 inch thick

Preparation
- Wash the carrots and cut into 1-inch-long pieces.
- Wash and core the apple, then cut into 1-inch pieces. Fill a dish with water and a few grains of sea salt and add the sliced apple to prevent it from oxidizing during the juice preparation.
- Place the carrots in a juicer and juice according to your juicer manufacturer's instructions, then do the same with the apple.
- Peel the orange, cut the wedges in half, and place in the juicer.
- Squeeze the lemon directly into the juice, then use a wooden utensil to stir.
- Mix well, then pour the juice into two glasses and enjoy immediately.

CARROT CELERY JUICE

Preparation time: 10 minutes
Serves 1

Ingredients
- 3 to 4 large carrots
- 1 to 1½ stalks celery

Preparation
- Wash the carrots and cut into 1-inch-long pieces.
- Wash the celery and cut into ½-inch pieces.
- Place the carrots in a juicer and juice according to your juicer manufacturer's instructions, then do the same with the celery.
- Pour the juice into a glass and enjoy immediately.

LEAFY GREENS JUICES

These juices are mildly sweet and slightly sour. Combining these two flavors relaxes the liver and the gallbladder. These juices are particularly helpful for a spring detox. Of course, you can enjoy them anytime you want a little extra lift.

While these juices might seem tame, they have a very powerful effect on your body. Because of this, we recommend a smaller serving size of these juices. Each juice recipe makes one serving, or half a cup of juice. Since different varieties of leafy greens yield different amounts of juice, I find it helpful to juice directly into a liquid measuring cup, and have specified the ingredients as such. This way you will know exactly how much juice each ingredient yields.

SWEET DREAM OF GREEN (NAPA, GREEN APPLE, CABBAGE)

Preparation time: 10 minutes
Serves 1

Ingredients
- ⅛ cup napa cabbage juice, approximately 2 to 3 leaves napa
- ⅛ cup green head cabbage juice, approximately 1 cup cabbage
- ¼ cup green apple, approximately ½ green apple

Preparation
- Wash and cut the green cabbage into 1-inch pieces.
- Wash and cut the napa cabbage into 1-inch pieces.

- Wash and cut the apple in half. Core one of the halves and cut into 1-inch pieces. Refrigerate the other half in a sealed dish with a little water and a squeeze of fresh lemon juice.
- Place the green head cabbage in a juicer and juice according to your juicer manufacturer's instructions, then do the same with the napa, then the apple.
- Pour the juice in a glass and enjoy immediately.

COOL GREEN CUCUMBER JUICE
(NAPA, CUCUMBER, GREEN APPLE)

Preparation time: 10 minutes
Serves 1

Ingredients
- ¼ cup fresh napa cabbage juice, approximately 3 to 4 leaves napa
- ⅛ cup fresh green apple juice, approximately ½ green apple
- ⅛ cup cucumber juice, approximately ¼ to ⅓ cucumber

Preparation
- Wash and cut the leafy greens into 1-inch pieces.
- Wash and cut the cucumber into 1-inch pieces.
- Wash and cut the apple in half. Core and cut into 1-inch pieces. Store the other half in the refrigerator.

- Place the napa in a juicer and juice according to your juicer manufacturer's instructions, then do the same with the green apple and the cucumber.
- Pour the juice in a glass and consume immediately.

GREEN TWIST

Ingredients
- ⅛ cup green cabbage juice
- ⅛ cup cucumber juice, ¼ to ⅓ cucumber
- ¼ cup bok choy juice, approximately 2 to 3 leaves bok choy
- A few sprigs of fresh parsley, approximately ⅛ cup parsley juice
- 1 wedge fresh lemon

Preparation
- Wash and cut the cabbage into 1-inch pieces.
- Wash and cut the bok choy into 1-inch pieces.
- Wash the parsley.
- Wash and cut the cucumber into 1-inch pieces.
- Place the green cabbage in a juicer and juice according to your juicer manufacturer's instructions, then do the same with the bok choy, then the parsley, then the cucumber.
- Squeeze fresh lemon directly into the greens juice and stir.
- Pour the juice into a glass and enjoy immediately.

10-DAY MENU PLAN

Here is menu for ten days of macrobiotic eating. If you are new to this way of eating, try just a few days and see how you feel. If you're feeling good, then try the whole ten days. If you love how you feel and want to continue, this menu is designed so that you can go right back to day one. Keep in mind that when making changes to your diet, you might feel a little strange for a few days until your body adjusts to this new way of eating.

ADDING VARIETY:

When you repeat this menu plan every 10 days, feel free to change the vegetables used in the recipes to include more variety in your diet. For example, bok choy, mustard greens, and collards are all excellent substitutes for kale. Also feel free to explore the other recipes included in this book.

GLUTEN-FREE OPTIONS:

I have given some optional grain dishes and substitutions for those who follow a gluten-free diet. If you are gluten-free, substitute Gluten-Free Tamari for any shoyu seasoning, and use brown rice miso instead of aged barley miso.

DAY 1

Breakfast
- Millet with Sweet Vegetables: onion and cauliflower
- Quick Steamed Greens with Fresh-Squeezed Lemon

Lunch
- Brown Rice with Pearled Barley or Brown Rice with Hato Mugi Barley (GF)
- Miso Soup: aged barley miso, wakame sea vegetable, dried shiitake mushrooms, daikon radish, napa cabbage, finely chopped scallion garnish
- Sweet Vegetable Kinpira: carrot, onions, parsnip
- Blanched Vegetable Salad: bok choy, broccoli, red radish. Serve with a few drops of brown rice vinegar.

Mid-Afternoon Snack
- Fresh carrot juice or carrot-combination juice

Dinner
- Farro with White beans and Kale or Peruvian Quinoa Salad with Black Beans (GF)
- Steamed Sweet Potato
- Fresh Arugula Salad with Tofu Cheese
- Poached Pear in Balsamic Barley Malt Reduction

DAY 2

Breakfast
- Soft Rice: use leftover rice from yesterday's lunch and season with umeboshi plum, garnish with a half sheet of toasted nori if desired
- Blanched Vegetable Salad: napa cabbage, broccoli, carrots

Lunch

- Leftover Farro or Quinoa
- Miso Soup: sweet-tasting brown rice miso, wakame sea vegetable, onion, turnip, turnip greens or other leafy greens, scallion garnish
- Leftover Kinpira from Day 1
- Quick Steamed Leafy Greens with Fresh Lemon

Mid-Afternoon Snack

- Leftover steamed sweet potato or leafy greens juice

Dinner

- Pan-fried Millet Croquettes: use the leftover millet from Day 1 breakfast, add a little cornmeal to thicken, form into patties and pan-fry on medium-low heat until cooked through.
- Vegan Tartar Sauce: mix together two tablespoons tahini, 2 tablespoons freshly-grated daikon radish, ¼ teaspoon shoyu, ½ teaspoon green nori flakes
- Savory French Lentils with Onions, Leeks, and Fresh Herbs
- Asian-Style Leafy Greens
- Quick Umeboshi Vinegar Pickles: use red cabbage
- Fresh Fruit Kanten

DAY 3

Breakfast

- Steel Cut Oats with Maple Syrup
- Blanched Vegetable Salad: green cabbage, collards, carrots

Lunch

- Brown Rice with Sweet Brown Rice: garnish with lightly toasted chopped walnuts

- Miso Soup: aged barley miso, wakame sea vegetable, dried maitake mushroom, lotus root, onion, and watercress
- Leftover lentils from Day 2
- Quick Sautéed Vegetables: red onion, bok choy and carrots

Mid-Afternoon Snack
- Fresh Carrot Juice or Carrot Combination Juice

Dinner
- Fried Noodles: use wheat or gluten-free noodles
- Nishime Vegetables: use sweet root and round vegetables like sweet potato, cabbage, onion
- Fresh Salad: hearts of romaine lettuce, cucumbers, pickled red onion, vinaigrette dressing
- Amasake kanten

DAY 4

Breakfast
- Leftover Steel Cut Oats: top with ume-shiso sprinkle
- Quick Steamed greens

Lunch
- Vegetable Sushi: use the leftover brown rice and sweet rice from Day 3. Fill with fried tempeh special sauce, sauerkraut, blanched carrots, and cucumber; or cucumber, fresh shiso leaves, umeboshi paste.
- Susan's Special Sushi Sauce: mix together 1 part roasted tahini, 1 part umeboshi paste, and 1 part mustard. Add a small amount of wasabi powder if desired and thin to desired consistency with water.
- Cream of Broccoli Leek Soup: garnish with fresh herbs
- Leftover Nishime

- Quick Sautéed Leafy Greens: bok choy, baby bok choy, olive oil

Mid-Afternoon Snack
- Warm Apple Cider with Fresh Lemon

Dinner
- Couscous with Sautéed Vegetables or Quinoa with Sautéed Vegetables (GF)
- White Beans with Cabbage and Caraway
- Mediterranean-Style Cauliflower
- Fresh Arugula Salad with Tofu Cheese
- Red Grape Fresh Fruit Kanten

DAY 5

Breakfast
- Steamed Sourdough Bread or Gluten Free Bread with apple butter or other spread
- Blanched Vegetable Salad: cabbage, kale, and red radish

Lunch
- Leftover Couscous or Quinoa
- Leftover White Beans and Cabbage
- Quick Steamed Greens: collard greens with fresh lemon
- Quick Umeboshi Vinegar Pickles

Mid-Afternoon Snack
- Fresh Carrot Juice or Carrot Combination Juice

Dinner
- Brown Rice with Wild Rice: top with toasted sunflower or sesame seeds
- Leftover Creamy Soup: with fresh herb garnish

- Sautéed Watercress with Asian seasoning
- Fresh Salad: hearts of romaine, iceberg lettuce, cucumber, radicchio, tofu cheese
- Leftover Grape Kanten

DAY 6

Breakfast
- Soft corn grits: make extra grits, pour into a Pyrex dish, and use on Day 7
- Blanched Vegetable Salad: cauliflower, collards, red radish or daikon radish

Lunch
- Fried Rice: use leftover rice
- Miso Soup: aged barley miso, wakame sea vegetable, turnips, turnip greens, chopped scallion garnish
- Arame with Onions, Carrots, Fresh Tofu
- Quick Steamed Greens with Fresh Lemon

Mid-Afternoon Snack
- Warm amasake, slightly diluted with water

Dinner
- Penne Pasta: sautéed broccoli rabe and sun-dried tomatoes
- White Beans with Sautéed Escarole
- Fresh Salad: arugula, pickled red radish, steamed beets, toasted pine nuts
- Fresh Berries with Almond Creme

DAY 7

Breakfast
- Soft Rice

- Water-Sautéed Watercress

Lunch
- Pan-Fried Polenta: use the extra polenta you made at breakfast yesterday
- Leftover White Beans
- Blanched Vegetable Salad: napa cabbage, string beans, summer squash, and carrots
- Quick Umeboshi Vinegar Pickles

Mid-Afternoon Snack
- Fresh Leafy Greens Juice

Dinner
- Brown Rice with Lentils and Sautéed Onions
- Miso Soup: aged barley miso, wakame sea vegetable, dried shiitake mushrooms, daikon radish, and leafy greens
- Leftover Arame
- Quick Steamed Greens with fresh lemon
- Baked Apple: with toasted walnuts and currents

DAY 8

Breakfast
- Rolled Oats with Umeboshi Plum
- Quick Steamed Greens

Lunch
- Fried Tempeh Wrap: spread an organic steamed wrap with tahini and top with sautéed onions and mushrooms, fried tempeh, and lettuce
- Red Bean Soup with Fresh Herb Garnish
- Sautéed Cauliflower
- Quick Umeboshi Vinegar Pickles: red cabbage

Mid-Afternoon Snack
- Fresh Carrot Juice or Carrot Combination Juice

Dinner
- Leftover Brown Rice with Lentils
- Miso Soup: sweet-tasting brown rice miso, wakame sea vegetable, onion, turnip, tofu cubes, leafy greens, scallion garnish
- Candied Sweet Potatoes
- Arugula Salad with Sautéed Mushrooms
- Leftover Baked Apple

DAY 9

Breakfast
- Sweet Couscous
- Blanched Vegetable Salad: green cabbage, kale, carrots

Lunch
- Brown Rice with Quinoa
- Leftover Candied Sweet Potatoes
- Quick Sautéed Leafy Greens

Mid-Afternoon Snack
- Fresh Leafy Greens Juice

Dinner
- Italian-Style Pasta with Cauliflower Sauce
- Red Bean Soup
- Quick Steamed Greens with Fresh Lemon
- Panna Cotta

DAY 10

Breakfast
- Soft Millet with Sweet Vegetables
- Water-Sautéed Watercress

Lunch
- Fried Udon Noodles
- Miso Soup: aged barley miso, wakame sea vegetable, onion, lotus root, celery greens, scallion garnish
- Roots and Greens
- Blanched Vegetable Salad: napa, broccoli, red radish served with brown rice vinegar

Dinner
- Leftover Brown Rice with Quinoa
- Steamed Corn Tortillas, with sautéed onions and mushrooms
- Refried Beans
- Fried Parsnip Chips
- Vegan Caesar Salad with Avocado
- Fresh Seasonal Fruits or Steamed Fruit

HEALTHFUL FOODS LIST

FOODS FOR REGULAR USE

These are the most important foods for everyone.
They are essential to a healthful, balanced, and nutritious diet.

GRAINS AND GRAIN PRODUCTS

Use a variety with every meal. Eat brown rice often or daily.

WHOLE GRAINS	WHOLE, CRACKED & FLAKED GRAINS	FLOUR PRODUCTS
Use often	*Use occasionally*	*Use occasionally*
Short-grain brown rice	Sweet brown rice	Whole-wheat noodles
Medium-grain brown rice	Pounded sweet rice (Mochi)	Italian pasta (organic)
Barley (hulled)	Hato-mugi barley,	Gluten-free pasta
Barley (pearled)	Pearl barley, Job's tears,	Japanese wheat noodles
Millet	Barley grits	(Udon)
Wheat berries	Bulgur	Japanese thin wheat
Farro	Cracked wheat	noodles (Somen)
Corn (corn-on-the-cob)	Couscous	Japanese buckwheat
Whole oats	Rolled oats	noodles (Soba)
Rye	Steel cut oats	Bread: un-yeasted,
Buckwheat	Corn grits	sourdough,
Long grain brown rice	Cornmeal (Polenta)	Whole-wheat, spelt or rye
(for hot climates)	Rye flakes, barley flakes	Puffed wheat gluten (Fu)
	or other flakes	Boiled wheat gluten (Seitan)
	Other traditional grains	
	including amaranth, quinoa,	
	teff, etc.	

VEGETABLE SOUPS

1 to 2 servings every day with a meal

Mildly season soups with barley miso, brown rice miso, shoyu, or sea salt.
Use barley (mugi) miso or brown rice (genmai) miso.
Garnish soups often with chopped scallion or parsley.

Miso vegetable soup—with wakame seaweed, a variety of vegetables, dried shiitake occasionally and miso.

Puréed sweet vegetable soup—seasoned with sea salt or shoyu.

Puréed sweet vegetable soup with millet or barley—Cook in a small amount of leftover grain to make a creamy soup. Season with sea salt or shoyu.

Other types of vegetable soup—with a variety of vegetables, sea vegetables, beans, grains or pasta.

Bean vegetable soup—Cook leftover beans in vegetable soup until creamy.

Grain vegetable soup—Cook leftover grains such as brown rice, barley, or millet in vegetable soup until creamy. Season with miso or shoyu.

Noodle vegetable soup—with wheat or buckwheat noodles.

Fish vegetable soup—with white meat fish.

VEGETABLES

Eat one or more vegetable dishes with every meal.

Do not reheat leftover vegetable dishes; take them out and let them warm up naturally

Use often	Use Often	Use occasionally
[1] Green Leafy:	**[3] Root:**	Arugula
Bok choy	Burdock	Broccoli rabe
Carrot tops	Carrots	Celery
Chinese cabbage (napa)	Daikon	Chives
Collard greens	Dandelion roots	Cucumber
Daikon greens	Jinenjo (yamaimo)	Endive
Dandelion greens	Lotus root	Escarole
Kale	Parsnip	Green beans
Leek	Radish	Green peas
Mustard greens		Iceberg lettuce
Parsley	**[4] Sweet vegetables:**	Jerusalem artichoke
Scallion	Sweet vegetables are a combination of round and root vegetables. These vegetables become sweet when cooked *Broccoli and cauliflower are not usually considered sweet vegetables, however, they add a richness and freshness to puréed soups when combined with the sweet vegetables.	Kohlrabi
Turnip greens		Lambsquarters
Watercress		Mushrooms
[2] Round:		Patty pan squash
Acorn squash		Purslane
Broccoli		Romaine lettuce
Brussels sprouts		Salsify
Buttercup squash		Snap beans
Butternut squash	Broccoli*	Snow peas
Cabbage	Cabbage	Sprouts
Cauliflower	Carrots	Summer squash
Hokkaido pumpkin	Cauliflower*	Wax beans
Onion	Daikon	
Pumpkin	Leek	
Red cabbage	Onion	
Rutabaga	Parsnip	
Turnip	Pumpkin	
Shiitake mushroom (dried)	Sweet potato	
Maitake	Winter Squash	

BEANS AND BEAN PRODUCTS

Use beans or bean products at one or two meals a day.

Cook beans with a 1-inch piece of kombu seaweed to make them more digestible. Beans may be also served with a teaspoon of grated daikon with a dash of shoyu. Beans may be cooked with vegetables, with grains, or in soups. Season beans at the end of cooking with sea salt or shoyu.

BEANS	BEANS	BEAN PRODUCTS*
Use often	*Use occasionally*	*Use occasionally*
Azuki beans	Black-eyed peas	Fresh tofu
Black soybeans	Black turtle beans	Dried tofu
Chickpeas-Garbanzos	Cannellini beans	Natto
Green or black lentils	Great Northern beans	Edamame
	Kidney beans	Tempeh
	Lima beans	
	Mung beans	
	Navy beans	
	Pinto beans	
	Soybeans*	
	Split peas	
	Whole dried peas	

*Organic, non-GMO

SEA VEGETABLES

Use small amounts daily in cooking.

Nori, wakame, and kombu are used as a part of daily cooking.
They are used in a variety of dishes including: soups, vegetable, bean, and grain
dishes.

Use often	*Use occasionally*	*Optional use:*
Toasted nori sheet	Arame (as a side dish)	Agar-agar
Wakame	Hiziki (as a side dish)	Dulse
Kombu		Irish Moss

PICKLED VEGETABLES

Use as a garnish almost daily.

A small amount of natural sauerkraut and other natural pickles can be used.
Wash or soak the pickles if they taste salty.

Use often	*Use occasionally*
Pressed pickles	Bran or miso-bran pickles
Sauerkraut	Daikon radish pickles (Takuan)
Quick ume-vinegar pickles	Miso or shoyu pickles
Brine pickles	
Kimchi	

TABLE CONDIMENTS

Try to use 1-2 condiments every day

Condiments are used on foods at the table—not in cooking.
Make a condiment tray and keep it on the table as a reminder to use them.
Condiments with an (*) can be bought; it is best to make the others at home.

Use often	*Use occasionally*
Sesame Salt (Gomashio): ½-1 tsp.	Scallion miso condiment: 1-2 tsp.
Toasted sesame seeds: 1-2 tsp.	Tekka (Root vegetable and miso
Green Ao nori flakes*: ½-1 tsp.	condiment)*: ¼ tsp.
Shiso powder-sprinkle*: ¼ tsp.	Brown rice vinegar*: 4-5 drops
Umeboshi plums* (Ryujin): ½-1 plum	Lemon juice
Umeboshi vinegar*: 4-5 drops	Apple Cider vinegar

SEASONINGS FOR COOKING

Use the full variety to make your food tasty.

Seasonings are used in cooking—not at the table.

Use often	*Use occasionally*
Unrefined white sea salt (Si brand)	Brown rice vinegar
Barley miso (Mugi): aged at least 2 years	Apple Cider vinegar
Brown rice miso (Genmai): aged at least	Ginger
1 year	Horseradish
Shoyu (naturally fermented soy sauce)	Wasabi horseradish
Light sesame oil	Umeboshi plum
Extra virgin olive oil	Umeboshi paste
	Umeboshi vinegar
	Garlic
	Lemon
	Soybean miso (Hatcho)
	Mirin (sweet taste)
	Toasted/dark sesame oil
	European herbs

BEVERAGES

Drink a comfortable amount for thirst.

Use often	*Use occasionally*	*Use occasionally*
Bancha twig tea-kukicha	Pure grain coffee	Black coffee or tea
Roasted barley tea	Bancha leaf tea-green tea	Carrot or carrot-greens juice
Roasted brown rice tea	Dandelion tea	Carrot, apple, and greens
Filtered water (carbon	Kombu tea	juice
block)	Mu tea (mild)	Carrot, apple, and orange
		juice
		Micro-brewed beer
		Natural sake
		Red or white wine
		Sweet vegetable drink

FOODS FOR OCCASIONAL USE

Quite a number of people who are practicing macrobiotics today are also choosing to go vegan and not include fish. This way of eating is easily adaptable to a vegan diet while also providing complete nutrition.

FISH

1 to 3 times a week

Carp	Red Snapper
Cod	Scrod
Flounder	Sole
Haddock	Other non-fatty, white-meat fish
Halibut	Salmon

SEEDS AND NUTS

1 to 2 cups seeds, and 1 to 2 cups nuts a week (lightly roasted, unsalted)

Seeds and nuts may be used in cooking, as garnishes with a variety of dishes, and as snacks.
Seeds and nuts may be eaten boiled, blanched, lightly dry, or oil-roasted.
Pumpkin seeds and occasionally sunflower seeds and walnuts may be eaten raw.

Seeds

Pumpkin seeds
Sesame seeds
Sunflower seeds
Roasted tahini

Nuts

Chestnuts
Almonds
Peanuts
Walnuts
Pecans
Peanut butter
Other nut butters

SNACKS

Can be used almost daily

Snacks may be eaten in moderate amounts.
Try not to let them interfere with your regular meals.

Leftovers
Pounded sweet rice (Mochi)
Noodles
Nuts
Seeds

Puffed whole cereal grains
Popcorn-homemade,
unbuttered
Rice cakes
Rice balls
Corn Thins

Sweet vegetable jam
Nori, brown rice, and
vegetables
(Sushi)

SWEETS AND SWEETENERS

Can be used almost daily

Use often

Sweet vegetables
Sweet vegetable drink
Sweet vegetable ham
Chestnuts or chestnut purée

Use occasionally

Amasake
Barley malt (pure)
Brown rice syrup
Pure maple syrup
Hot apple cider: diluted with bancha twig tea or filtered water
Hot apple juice: diluted with bancha twig tea or filtered water

FRUITS

3 to 7 times a week

Cooked or fresh, seasonal Northern climate fruits

Seeds

Blueberries
Cantaloupe
Honeydew
Raspberries
Strawberries
Watermelon

Tree Fruit

Apples
Apricots
Cherries
Grapes
Peaches
Pears
Plums
Tangerines
Oranges

USE SPARINGLY OR AVOID

These foods depend on your health.
Many are very acidifying or affect blood sugar.

BAKED FLOUR PRODUCTS AND REFINED GRAINS

Muffins
Crackers
Cookies
Pancakes
Chips
Baked pastries
White rice

BEVERAGES

Green magma
Northern climate fruit juices
Whiskey (natural quality)
Soy milk (with kombu)
Rice Dream beverage
Rice Milk
Frozen Rice Dream

SEASONINGS AND SPICES

All spices
All commercial seasonings
All herbs

VEGETABLES

Artichoke
Asparagus
Avocado
Bamboo shoots
Beets
Curly dock
Eggplant
Fennel
Ferns
Ginseng
Green or red pepper
New Zealand spinach
Okra
Plantain
Potato
Rhubarb
Spinach
Tomato (fresh or sun-dried)
Taro potato (albi)
Yam
Zucchini

PICKLES

Dill pickles
Herb pickles
Garlic pickles
Spiced pickles
Vinegar pickles
Apple cider vinegar pickles
Wine vinegar pickles

BLUE-SKINNED FISH

Herring
Sardines

ALL TROPICAL NUTS

Brazil nuts
Cashews
Hazel nuts
Macadamia nuts
Pistachio nuts

ALL TROPICAL FRUIT, INCLUDING:

Dates
Figs
Mango
Papaya
Pineapple
Grapefruit

AVOID AS MUCH AS POSSIBLE

These are the worst foods for everybody.

RED MEAT

Beef
Lamb
Pork

POULTRY

Chicken
Duck
Turkey

BLUE-SKINNED FISH

Tuna
Bluefish
Swordfish

DAIRY FOODS

Milk
Butter
Yogurt
Frozen yogurt
Ice cream

BEVERAGES

Artificial beverages
Cold drinks, iced drinks
Distilled water
Hard liquor
Herbal teas
Mineral-bubbling waters
Regular tea
Stimulant beverages
Sugared beverages
Tap water
Carbonated waters

SWEETENERS

Agave nectar
Artificial sweeteners
Brown sugar
Carob
Chocolate
Corn sugar
High-fructose corn syrup
Concentrated fruit
sweeteners
Honey
Molasses
Stevia
Sugar substitutes
White sugar

OTHER FOODS

Bananas
Coconut
Coconut oil
Lard
Margarine
Artificially processed foods
All foods containing trans
fats

STYLES OF COOKING

Use often	Use occasionally
Pressure cooking	Baking
Boiling	Broiling
Blanching	Dry roasting
Steaming	Pan-frying
Steaming with kombu (Nishime)	Deep frying
Soup making	Tempura (batter dipped and deep fried)
Stewing	
Quick water sautéeing	
Quick oil sautéeing	
Sautéeing & simmering (Kimpira)	
Sautéeing	
Pickling	
Raw	

FOOD GLOSSARY

The goal was to keep these recipes simple. Wherever possible, we have used familiar ingredients. We understand that any change in diet requires a rethinking of old food habits; having to learn about new food products presents an additional challenge. You will find, however, that many of the recipes do include unfamiliar ingredients, products that have such strong health benefits and are so delicious that it is important to become familiar with them and use them on a regular basis. The following is a list of some of those items:

Jinenjo/Yamaimo: Sometimes referred to as "Japanese mountain yam". A strong root vegetable that grows in the mountains. Jinenjo aids digestion and strengthens vitality. Jinenjo is usually grated raw, with toasted nori, chopped scallions, and shoyu. Typically served with a sauce over rice or noodles, or in miso soup. Jinenjo can also be cooked like a potato in soups or stews. Usually available in Asian markets.

Miso: Miso is a remarkable food and is most beneficial when used as a seasoning for soup. Once you get into the habit of using it, you will wonder how you ever managed to cook without it. Miso is a paste made of fermented soybeans, grains, water, and sea salt. Miso is a valuable source of proteins, B vitamins, and minerals. Miso also contains enzymes that aid digestion and strengthen blood quality. Miso soup acts as an antidote to stress by relaxing the nervous system. There are many different types of miso from which to choose. The best kind for daily use is barley miso, also called mugi miso. The other is brown rice miso. Sweet white miso is lighter in taste and will add variety to your meals. Many more types of miso are available and it is fine to use other varieties occasionally; however, for optimum health use barley or brown rice miso on a regular basis. It is important to use only miso that is natural (traditionally made) and that has been aged for at least two years. Make sure to buy this product at a reputable health-food store.

Natto: A fermented soy product with a sticky texture and unusual odor. An acquired taste that makes you strong, brilliant, and beautiful. Natto strengthens digestion and vitality, cleans the skin, and clears the mind. It has unique qualities for strengthening the bones and for cleaning the cardiovascular system. Natto is eaten with rice, noodles, or in miso soup. It is prepared by mixing it with chopped scallions, toasted nori, mustard, and shoyu and mixed together until sticky.

Shiso leaves/Shiso powder: Another digestive aid, used as a condiment with grains or vegetables.

Shoyu: Everyone has used soy sauce, either at home or at a Chinese restaurant. Shoyu is simply traditionally made, naturally fermented soy sauce. What distinguishes it from regular soy sauce is the fact that it is not chemically processed. It is made from soybeans, wheat, sea salt, and water. Use shoyu with a light touch. Do not drown your food in it! Shoyu should be used only for cooking, not at the table. Keep it in the kitchen. Overuse leads to intense thirst and a strong craving for sweets. A small amount of shoyu goes a long way.

Umeboshi plums: Umeboshi is a salt-pickled plum that has both a sour and salty flavor. The red color of the plums comes from being pickled with shiso leaves. It aids digestion, strengthens blood quality, and is highly alkalizing. Umeboshi plum has the ability to neutralize the harmful effects caused by both animal foods and sugar. Umeboshi plum, or paste, is used to make sauces and dressings and is delicious on corn on-the-cob.

Umeboshi vinegar: This vinegar is extracted from the Japanese ume plum. Sorry, I know we promised to keep it simple, but this vinegar is so delicious and so taste-enhancing that we thought you should become familiar with it. The use of umeboshi vinegar will help lighten your digestion.

Udon noodles: These are Japanese wheat noodles. They have a nice light flavor and are free of chemical preservatives.

Sea Salt: Sea salt is evaporated from sea water and washed. We recommend unrefined and white sea salts. High-quality sea salt has a soft, mildly sweet taste before tasting salty. High-quality sea salt is as essential for health as it is for taste.

Sea Vegetables: kombu and wakame: Sea vegetables are the plants of the sea. They are packed with vitamins, minerals, and trace elements. Sea vegetables are further protective against heavy metals, pollutants, and radioactivity. They are cooked in small quantities in soups or with vegetables and beans.

We hope that you found this section helpful and that you enjoy using these ingredients. Once you become familiar with the ingredients, you will find it easy to improvise and come up with variations of your own.

Good health is built on the choices we make daily. Don't forget, every day, at every meal, make sure to have both a grain and a separate vegetable dish. Take one or two small bowls of vegetable soup daily. You will be amazed at how much better you will feel.